Natural PAINKILLERS

Without *Drug Dependence or Side Effects*

By
James W. Forsythe, M.D., H.M.D.

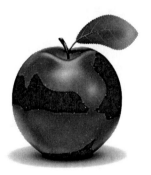

Natural PainKillers

Century Wellness Publishing

Copyright © 2012, By James W. Forsythe, M.D., H.M.D.

All Rights Reserved, including the right of reproduction in whole or in part in any form. This is a first edition.

Forsythe, James W., M.D., H.M.D.

Book Design: Patty Atcheson Melton

1. Health   2. Diets

ISBN: 978-0-9848383-7-0

DEDICATION

To my entire office staff, including my wife, Earlene, an administrator and an Advanced Nurse Practitioner (A.P.N.), office manager Valerie Kilgore, R.N., and my two associates, Dr. Maged Maged, and Dr. Samuel Winter.

I also dedicate this book to all my patients, alive and deceased, who have bravely suffered through severe and incapacitating pains of all imaginable types. Hopefully, this book will help assist my current and future patients in using natural therapies to eliminate and inactivate these symptoms, either used alone or coupled with conventional medications.

FOREWARD

Every day worldwide hundreds of thousands of people suffer from needless pain because they rely on the reckless advice of physicians that prescribe dangerous drugs.

This generates a proverbial double-edged sword. Countless patients develop debilitating addictions to extremely harmful prescription painkillers. Compounding the problem multi-fold, these dangerous substances often fail to alleviate the patients' underlying pain, while also occasionally generating serious complications.

All along, the vast majority of standard allopathic doctors who attend traditional medical schools hide a significant "secret" from the general public.

Namely, the mainstream medical industry strives to prevent consumers from learning about the vast availability of harmless, inexpensive natural substances that eliminate pain.

These plant-based herbs and minerals generated in abundance by Mother Nature never cause any adverse symptoms or negative side effects.

All along, while striving to avoid "natural pain cures" or even to inform the public that such options exist, the world's top-selling pharmaceutical companies generated $643 billion in 2006, a total that was likely to surpass $1 trillion in coming years.

These calculations listed in a variety of news reports including an article in "Forbes" magazine failed to pinpoint the underlying cause of this ballooning trend.

Well, as you'll soon discover in the pages that follow, everything comes down to two words—"greed" and "heartlessness."

Standard doctors are recklessly disregarding the need to protect the public's health, encouraged by greedy drug firms, bloated hospital bureaucracies and the related money-hungry health care businesses that they serve.

Meantime these same standard medicine physicians strive to badmouth the reputations of homeopathic doctors who champion the urgent need for natural pain cures.

Eager to satisfy steadily increasing public demand for the truth, this publication contains streams of easy-to-understand details describing a vast array of natural cures.

What are the best natural remedies for specific painful ailments, everything from headaches to backaches? Where can consumers get such products at a low, fair and reasonable price? Just as important, what potentially fraudulent "natural" substances are on the market, and how can patients detect such schemes?

With just as much fervor, "Natural Pain Cures" also delves deep into the urgent and overriding need for patients to ask their standard-medicine doctors critical questions.

Indeed, patients suffering from a wide range of ailments spanning from arthritis to leg cramps should learn how to push their doctors for "natural, harmless options."

While focusing on the best overall strategy for consumers, patients also learn of the many misconceptions about pain. As readers will soon discover, a bogus, unhealthy and needless age-old saying proclaims "no pain, no gain."

To the contrary, however, excessive and unnecessary pain can and often does lead to debilitating lifelong health challenges in some patients. The biggest losers in this regard often emerge as those who strive to "fight through the pain," essentially exercising, competing or living everyday life without attempting to address the underlying health issues that cause extreme physical discomfort.

As if these many problems weren't already bad enough, in

many instances the standard medical industry requires physicians to prescribe ineffective, unhealthful or ineffective treatments ranging from chemotherapy to radiation. These treatments in the long run sometimes actually cause physical pain and even death.

Needless to say, as an integrative medical oncologist licensed in homeopathy and practicing standard medicine as well, I felt a burning desire to bring the cold, hard facts to the public here.

Many health care professionals, particularly homeopathic doctors who specialize in natural remedies, openly express their anger at the mainstream medical industry and the U.S. federal Food and Drug Administration for subjecting to the public to these needless dangers.

Although this book was not written as, nor was it intended to be, a religious publication, lots of patients appreciate the fact that the Book of John in the Holy Bible, in Chapter 8, Verse 32 says, "The truth shall set you free."

Such faith helps bring great hope to patients eager to escape the shackles imposed upon them by standard physicians who knowingly or unwittingly seek to enslave patients with extremely harmful and unnatural painkillers.

Taking a completely opposite approach, through my practice assisting cancer patients and people with a wide variety of other ailments, the "natural" options for addressing pain become my first and foremost options when addressing such symptoms.

Along the way, many patients are also amazed to discover that in some instances pain can actually be "an extremely good thing for them"—the reasons revealed in subsequent pages.

Even when such cases occur, patients often find comfort in learning from me or from my highly trained medical staff that numerous herbal products—either alone or in combination with various other natural substances—often serve as valuable options in the treatment of people who have suffered from mild to moderate pain.

Adding to the luster, readers also discover a vast array of minerals helpful for relieving the extremely uncomfortable physical sensations caused by numerous medical conditions, ranging from musculoskeletal injuries to arthritis.

Giving patients additional reason for hope, I also eagerly provide them with the positive news that an estimated 90 percent of all physical pains are highly treatable—particularly with natural substances rather than expensive and dangerous drugs.

Quite predictably, upon learning these details lots of patients eventually begin wondering, "Why should I endanger my health, when natural substances can handle the task just as well or perhaps even better than highly expensive, unnatural and addictive drugs generated by huge pharmaceutical companies? Where and how can I obtain the services of a homeopath that can help put me on a pathway toward natural painkillers? What would that cost, which of these expenses would insurance cover if any, and how do all these various critical factors compare with services, fees and drugs offered by standard doctors?"

Ultimately, as many of my patients discover to their great delight, the answers often are surprising and likely to generate positive responses among consumers.

--James W. Forsythe, M.D., H.M.D.

INTRODUCTION

Are You A Slave To Pain And Painkillers?

"God whispers to us in our pleasures, speaks to us in our conscience, but shouts in our pain: it is His megaphone to rouse a deaf world."

--C.S. Lewis

Pain is an equal opportunity condition. It can afflict anyone at anytime. It can arise from an injury, from an illness, a disease, from the wear and tear of advancing age, or it can spring forth fully felt from the deepest recesses of the human imagination. At some point in their life, about one-third of everyone in the U.S. will experience chronic pain, which is the most common cause of long term disability.

You may not realize that pain begins and ends in your mind. It's your brain that receives, translates and magnifies pain signals, whether you strained a muscle or burned a finger. It's your brain that's the center of these pain sensations and what pharmaceutical pain medications are formulated to do is to try and numb or interrupt the body's pain signals to the brain.

How we respond to the onset of physical pain plays a significant role in the eventual cessation of symptoms and sometimes provides a cure to an underlying problem. A timely response can make the difference between life and death, or the difference between a brief illness and a potential lifelong disability, because pain is telling you that damage is occurring to your body and you need to stop whatever you are doing that is causing the injury.

Those who ignore pain, or who flat-out refuse to seek a medical diagnosis of pain symptoms, can suffer a death that might have otherwise been prevented. Many people and their relatives often learn too late that those severe chest pains, jaw aches, headaches or backaches are the precursors to sudden though preventable fatalities.

You've heard the excuses and maybe you've used some of them yourself: "Oh, don't call an ambulance." Or they'll say, "We cannot afford the bills." Or they act dismissive with, "This must be just heartburn, or a hangover. Let's wait a little while and see if this thing passes."

Now entering my fifth decade as a full-time oncologist, I have seen countless cases where many people failed to heed the warning signs of pain—often until after it was too late to render effective treatment. On the positive side, many patients also quickly helped put themselves on track toward a return to vibrant health by visiting my office or the facilities of other medical professionals soon after their initial pain symptoms begin.

Untreated chronic and debilitating physical pain can also trigger the onset of severe depression. This mental condition affects all aspects of a person's life and further intensifies the overall experience of pain. Compounding the problem, some pharmaceutical drugs administered to combat pain can bring on a variety of mood disorders that, in a dangerous cycle, can result in even more drugs being prescribed with even more potential complications.

It's true that we've evolved a long way in our understanding of pain and the choice of methods we have at our disposal to treat it. During the 1950s surgeons commonly used lobotomies (partial nerve severing or removal of brain tissue) to numb severe pain. One famous victim of this practice was Argentina's Eva Peron (made more recently famous by Madonna in the movie, *Evita),* whose cervical cancer produced intense pain that was treated in 1952 with the brain surgery.

We are experiencing a pain occurrence problem and a pain medication abuse problem happening simultaneously in the U.S. and many other countries of the world. These problems have become intertwined. The more intense --and various-- levels of pain that we humans are forced to endure brings with it a frantic search for more powerful pain relievers and the attendant potential for physical damage, over use and abuse, and long term addiction.

Our over reliance on a pharmaceutical drug solution to treating pain has produced two huge unanticipated health consequences: life threatening side effects, and a widening cycle of drug dependency.

Life threatening side effects from some pharmaceutical pain medications have been well documented and widely publicized. Remember Celebrex, marketed for arthritis pain? Or who can forget Vioxx, or even Bextra, both eventually withdrawn from store shelves? They racked up billions of dollars in sales for the drug companies, but not only did these pain relief drugs fail to become the miracles that we were promised, we have since learned, in the words of Nutritional Biochemist Dr. Shawn M. Talbott, that "these drugs are no more effective at relieving pain than the aspirin in your medicine cabinet---and we know that they're killing thousands of us by causing heart attacks and stroke."

Even seemingly innocuous over the counter drugs such as

the brand names Aleve and Advil can have serious side effects—injuring your kidneys and stomach lining--- if you use them too often. So never take safety for granted since any drug you use to reduce pain may carry some risk to your health.

Today the problems with the more potent synthetic prescribed pain relievers have taken on a new dimension of concern with the spread of dependency. If we don't experience the pain pill abuse and addiction firsthand in our own lives or in the lives of people we care about, we usually hear about the effects of abuse most dramatically in sensational media headlines. During the 2011 trial of singer Michael Jackson's personal physician, for example, an addictions expert, Dr. Robert Waldman, testified that the pop star "was probably addicted to opioid painkillers {Demerol}... six weeks of high dose use would result in addiction in any of us." Once the headlines about Jackson's painkiller problem faded from the spotlight, we were left with less heralded but much more important stories about the ever spreading ravages of addiction to pain meds.

Glance over news stories from just the late 2011 period and you will see a disturbing pattern of how these abuses have brought misery to countless individuals and exacted a septic shock to our entire culture.

U.S. Painkiller Overdose Deaths Tripled

Fatal overdoses from OxyContin and Vicodin, mostly in men and middle-aged adults, tripled from 1999 to 2008, according to the U.S. Centers for Disease Control and Prevention. At least 15,000 people a year now die from painkillers and much of that total is a result of pill addiction. The highest rate of abuse was found in the state of Oklahoma.

More than five million people in the U.S. during 2009-2010 admitted to using dangerous pain relievers without a prescription, or simply because they enjoy the high that these drugs can produce.

Due mainly to painkiller overdoses, drug deaths now exceed car crash fatalities each year in the U.S., with one life being claimed very 14 minutes. This is an amazing statistic that shows we are all potential victims of this epidemic, especially when addicts get behind the wheel of motor vehicles. "The seeds of the problem were planted more than a decade ago," noted a *Los Angeles Times* investigation (Sept. 18, 2011), "by well-meaning efforts by doctors to mitigate suffering, as well as aggressive sales campaigns by pharmaceutical manufacturers."

This isn't just a problem limited to the United States. An August 2011 analysis in the *British Medical Journal* described how opioid prescribing and opioid related deaths have increased "especially rapidly" in parts of the United Kingdom, Canada and Australia. The International Narcotics Board further declares that "addiction to prescription opioids is a problem in almost all countries…the board has estimated that between 1.4 million and 1.9 million Germans are addicted to prescription drugs."

Addiction to Painkillers Spawns Crime Wave

Pharmacy robberies and property crimes are both out of control in some regions of the U.S. due to painkiller addicts trying to feed their habits. In one particularly brutal incident a 33-year-old pain pill addict, accompanied by his 30-year-old addict wife, murdered a pharmacist, a clerk, and two customers while robbing a Medford, N.Y. pharmacy in June 2011 of an estimated 11,000 hydrocodone pills. (Hydrocodone is the main ingredient in Vicodin.)

That tragic case illustrates just how desperate pain pill addicts are, such that even the ultimate crime of murder doesn't stop them from trying to forcibly obtain what they crave. In this instance, the primary drug stolen was a low level painkiller, but even with that low level the addictive properties are still very insidious and troubling.

Elsewhere in the nation, up to two-thirds of property theft crimes are committed by pain pill addicts. On Cape Cod, Mass., for instance, the number of burglaries and break-ins done to secure property to sell for narcotic pain pills have been doubling each year. Most addicts are searching for 30-milligram tablets of oxycodone with acetaminophen, known as Perc 30s, which sell for about $1 per milligram. A stolen flat-screen television usually ends up being traded for about 30 of these pills.

Infants Being Born Addicted to Painkillers

An investigation by a CNN reporting team, examining Florida state health records, found more than 600 babies born addicted to painkillers in just the first half of 2010 in south Florida. The babies got hooked while still in the womb because their mothers were chronic users of the pain meds while pregnant.

These babies went through all of the classic drug withdrawal symptoms of sweating, rapid breathing, irritability, even seizures. Most pregnant women with an addiction problem refuse to seek treatment out of a fear that their children will be taken away by state authorities and placed into foster care.

Prescription pain drug abuse, as characterized by the White House Office on Drug Control Policy, has become "our nation's fastest-growing drug problem." More than one-quarter of opioid painkiller users are already addicts, estimates the Physicians for Responsible Opioid Prescribing.

By far the most popular is OxyContin with nearly 7 million prescriptions written for it in 2010, 12 times more than Vicodin. OxyContin only won U.S. Food and Drug Administration approval in 1995, yet the drug quickly became the best selling painkiller because its manufacturer, Purdue Pharma, pushed a marketing campaign for physicians to prescribe it to treat everything from back pain to arthritic conditions. The drug's dark side soon emerged, commented *Fortune* magazine in November 2011, as physicians discovered "the patients would crash, needing more and higher doses. Patients who took moderate amounts for backaches or arthritis could find themselves hooked."

No matter how much self-control you may think you can exercise over your life, you are no match for resisting dependency if you become a chronic long term user of these powerful medications. That prospect should be reason enough for you to be reading this book, especially if you are experimenting to find pain relief solutions that work for you.

Ladders and Thresholds of Pain

How a physician views and prescribes a pain medicine is based on the concept of an ascending 'ladder of pain' and the patient's own pain threshold. You have rungs of drugs, doses, and number of pills, and also the time of use. Here is how it's supposed to work, both for you and for the physician.

Cancer pain, which I see on a daily basis, is steady, long lasting, not affected by sleep or rest. It can be low grade as with some soreness in the extremities, a lasting mild headache, or chest discomfort, pain with swallowing, and excruciating pain that requires prescriptions. Even with that severity, we try to use the lowest level of pain control you can get, like Vicodin, then gradually increase the dosage.

You should be climbing the ladder the slowly. You might then go to Percocet, or Tramadol, which doesn't have addictive potential. After Percocet you have a choice to go to 10 milligrams of oxycodone. You are going up both the drug ladder and the dose ladder. If oxycodone isn't enough to quell the pain, you might add ibprofin or Aleve to create a synergy of effects. After oxycodone you might advance to methadone. Hydromorphone is addictive and is the next rung of the ladder, in two or four milligram strength.

If the pain is severe enough, the highest rung of the ladder is morphine in its various forms, with dose, time intervals, and pill form options; there is also the liquid form, which can be absorbed quickly through the mouth or tongue.

Common side effects of pharmaceutical drug painkillers include constipation, dry mouth, a diminished appetite, slowing of motor skills and reactions, light headedness. Less common reactions are nausea, vomiting, feelings of paranoia, delusions and nightmares. Symptoms of addiction to painkillers include uncontrolled urges to continue the euphoric state, a loss of judgment about right and wrong, obsessive-compulsive feelings accompanied by sweating, jitteriness, anxiety, insomnia, jumbled thoughts, rambling speech, and a general disorientation.

Pain severity has its own ladder that varies from one person to another. For example, childbirth will be the most pain that many women will experience in a lifetime, so the birthing process might rank as a 10 on the ladder of severity, with all other experiences of pain compared to that on the pain ladder. Other people may have been wounded or burned in military combat, marking their top rung on the pain ladder against which everything else will be compared, while some fortunate people may only have a headache or a broken bone as markers for their maximum experience of a pain threshold.

Just as with the ladder of pharmaceutical drug use and the ladder of pain thresholds, there is a ladder of natural pain relief treatments that should be your first resort---with the synthetic drug ladder being your last resort--- to combat pain symptoms. I know that approach to pain turns traditional allopathic medicine on its head, so to speak, running contrary to the generally accepted practice of most physicians to reflexively prescribe a pharmaceutical for every ailment. But you deserve to know there are cheaper, effective, no-side effect options that are worth trying first before you embark on a drug taking spree.

Learn Your Natural Pain Relief Options

My motivation in writing this book was to provide you with useful information, combined with a sense of hope, about the entire range of pain relief options, from the most natural with no side effects to the potentially dangerous and powerful prescription medications with numerous possible side effects. My orientation as a physician tends toward the use of natural substances and techniques to whatever extent possible and whenever possible to treat the 'ladder of pain.'

There is also a health care cost consideration for me in writing this book. Both as individuals and as a society we need to lower our health care expenditures while continuing to develop the best possible treatments with the fewest risks for side effects or drug dependence. Sometimes it's not always possible to eliminate pain, whether with pharmaceutical drugs or natural approaches, but we can always manage pain and lessen it using a combination of natural strategies.

Within these pages you will discover essential techniques, many little-known, that cost almost nothing to put into action for short term or long term relief. Those who stand to benefit range from people severely debilitated by crippling arthritis to anyone suffering severe pains from cancer, chemotherapy side effects, kidney stones, childbirth labor, toothaches and a host of other ailments.

Throughout this book you'll learn time-tested for reducing the risk of becoming addicted to painkillers, particularly the opioids, or becoming victimized by their side effects. Many systems will be described to increase your prospects of putting your life back into a manageable order during bouts of pain. These include:

- **Mind control:** Techniques for relaxing the mind and body to lessen the impact of pain.
- **Natural substances:** Numerous natural substances such as herbs and food nutrients have proven highly effective in eliminating severe aches and pains.
- **Symptom prevention:** Unique, creative and little-known strategies for stopping potential pain dead in its tracks before it even has a chance to begin.

Long before the advent of today's standard pharmaceutical medicines, people from various ancient and tribal cultures around the world used effective pain-killing methods that are being re-discovered and their effectiveness affirmed by medical science laboratories. A key to avoiding the risks associated with standard drugs is to first employ one or a combination of these relatively safe, non-invasive methods for easing or preventing physical pain.

Some of the latest medical study findings about the origin and nature of pain and natural techniques for suppressing it may surprise you:

Did you know that about 300 candidate 'pain genes' have been identified as of 2011, determining how sensitive you are to pain signals and how responsive you will be to pain relief remedies?

Are you aware that an American Cancer Society review of dozens of 'guided imagery' studies found this mental technique to be effective for pain treatment?

Have you heard about how studies discovered that practicing yoga releases a hormone that is effective in reducing physical and psychological symptoms of chronic pain?

This is just a sampling of the cutting edge research I have compiled for you to utilize in your quest to subdue the ravages of a most unwelcome companion on your life's journey.

It will also be useful for you to know essential facts about the pain phenomenon and how it affects you, including exactly how and why this sensation occurs within your body. You will learn these details in Part One of this book. In Part Two, you will find everything you need to know about Big Pharma's pain solutions along with advice on how to avoid the twin traps of dependency and other side effects. Part Three of this book brings you details about the wide spectrum of Nature's pain treatments and how you can best use these benign tools.

Whether it is you or someone you love that is suffering from bouts of debilitating and life-wrecking pain, this book offers an uncomplicated recipe for a new lease on life. Pain should always be regarded as a symptom of something to be cured, not a condition to be endured. It should never be allowed to control your experience of what being alive has to offer.

With that in mind, read on to discover which pain relief options—or combinations of options--- may work best for you to provide relief.

Important Note To Readers

What follows in Part One amounts to a 'natural history' of pain and its role in the human experience of life.

Some of you may choose to skip this section and jump to Part Two, if you are eager for detailed information on natural pain relief solutions.

However, I do feel that Part One offers useful information providing an overview of your condition and a foundation for addressing your approach to treatment options.

PART ONE
Origins of Pain and Its Relief

Chapter 1
Pain Plays A Vital Role In Our Lives

"Pain is good because it's bad," Dr. Anne Louise Oaklander, a pain specialist once told NBC News. "And it's the badness, the unpleasantness; the horrible emotions that are evoked when we feel pain that make it work so well."

Some patients who suffer from severe limb injuries from car accidents tell physicians that the pain feels as if they're being stabbed with knives and needles. People who have been shot often describe the sensation that seemed as if getting stabbed by thunder bolts. These sensations become possible only because physical receptors connected to nerves throughout the body communicate the information to the spinal cord. From there, the information shoots up into the brain, the organ that actually gives us the sensation of "feeling pain."

When you stub your toe on furniture in a dark room during the middle of the night, the actual sensation of pain is not in your foot but inside your brain.

This remains a critical and essential point to remember, especially for anyone interested in counteracting or eliminating the uncomfortable sensations of pain.

A key to the process of your body's capacity to express the sensation of pain are peripheral nerves leading through the spinal cord. Peripheral nerves detect problems in essential areas of the body, including the skin, internal organs, muscles, joints and bones. The endings of peripheral nerves are extremely sensitive, capable of discerning between the subtle differences of touch, temperature variations, vibrations, pressures and severe injury.

Among the peripheral nerves are nociceptors that serve as the body's essential and vital sensory receptors that detect potentially severe internal damage or injuries. Physicians call this process "nociception," the important trigger of perceiving pain.

Like all mammals, humans would literally die unless we "possessed the ability to suffer" from physical pain. That sensation commands that we take action to address the problem.

All areas of the body except the face contain essential dorsal root ganglions, interconnected to the spinal nerve system and relaying sensory information to the brain. The information transmission process from the site of an injury or disease to the head amazes even experienced medical professionals.

The nerve endings within the face that detect pain are trigeminal ganglion, part of the fifth cranial nerves system. These nerves are essential in the eating, speaking, eye movement, and smelling processes. Anyone who has ever accidentally bitten his tongue while eating or been hit in the face has learned first-hand the super-sensitivity of this nerve system.

Your Brain Welcomes Sensations of Pain

After initial transmission from nociceptors, the nerve fibers within the spinal cord send the information about pain upward toward the brain. The dorsal horn serves as the location where peripheral nerves enter the spinal cord. In order to transmit their signals, the nerve fibers release neurotransmitters. These electrical signals strive to activate various nerve cells, which work to convey the information to the thalamus within the brain.

Located between the midbrain and the cerebral cortex, the thalamus works to regulate a variety of functions including sleep, consciousness and alertness. The thalamus also regulates or detects a sense of space, and various physical sensations including pain.

As soon as the thalamus receives communication about pain, it forwards this information to three separate areas of the brain:

- **The Somatosensory cortex:** Located in the upper center of the brain called the parietal lobe, this identifies and detects the degree and location of pain within the body.

- **Limbic system:** This consists of a set of various structures within the brain above the brain stem, which work together to elicit emotion regarding the pain signals.

- **The frontal lobe:** Sometimes referred to as the frontal cortex, this area is often referred to as the "thinking" part of the brain. It can assign "meaning" to signals of pain, while pondering—and eventually deciding—what actions to take.

Whenever possible, the brain also orders the body to begin producing natural pain killers called endorphins and enkephalins. Endorphins often generate pleasant natural sensations, released by the body when a person exercises, experiences love, enjoys orgasms, feels excitement, tastes spicy foods, or experiences physical pain.

When you suffer from a serious injury or disease, Mother Nature strives to make you feel the physical pain and to experience emotion that serves as a call to action—while also seeking to make you ponder possible solutions.

"If the mortality rate seems high we must realize that nature is a ruthless teacher," said William S. Burroughs, a 20th Century American novelist, poet and essayist. "There are no second chances in Mother Nature's survival course."

Three Primary Pain Remedies

A combination of modern technology, nature and age-old remedies give us three primary strategies or short-term fixes for addressing physical pain. They are:

- **Message blocking:** Various pharmaceuticals and natural products that work to block the nerve system's messaging system, preventing the brain from recognizing pain.

- **Health renewal:** Curing or fixing the body's area that has been wounded in accidents or attacks, or specific organs afflicted by disease, or the primary illness.

● **Mind control and prevention:** Training the mind to block perceptions of pain, or adopting lifestyles or physical devices that are likely to prevent or lessen the likelihood of painful conditions.

Huge segments of the medical profession are designed to bring out the best possible results in each of these strategies. Since pain or the lack of it plays an integral role in our health, significant emphasis is placed on these methods. By some estimates many hundreds of billions or perhaps trillions of dollars are spent yearly on pain-relief.

And yet amazingly, despite significant advances in the practice of medicine, physicians still lack a single cure-all method of preventing or eliminating physical pain. Even since early childhood, many of us began hearing that common phrase, "there is no cure for the common cold." But few people pay attention to the fact medicine also lacks a single, reliable and predictably effective, non-addictive cure for excruciating physical pain.

In matters involving pain some people embrace and adhere to the longstanding lifestyle theme that "ignorance is bliss," since the mere thought of suffering with—and the seeking remedies for—severe pain seems extremely difficult or even insurmountable.

Most Physical Pain is Manageable

Most cases of pain are short-term and easily medicated. Almost everyone has suffered from common everyday cuts, bruises, sprains, blisters, headaches and joint aches. Remember that pain hails as a basic fact of life, and to satisfy the public's need to address minor afflictions, pharmaceutical and medical supply companies have developed a plethora of materials and over-the-counter drugs.

According to some estimates, the average American family spends about $185 yearly on non-prescription remedies. This brings the nationwide total for such purchases to many tens of billions of dollars.

The overall dollar totals catapult to far greater levels when accounting for prescription medications that only licensed doctors can legally administer, at least when distribution is handled on a domestic basis. Estimates vary widely, partly because significant numbers of Americans strive to buy pharmaceuticals cheaply online from international suppliers, rather than pay exorbitant U.S. prices.

The failure of the medical industry to develop a single affordable, reliable and predictable method of eliminating severe pain has played a primary role in driving up prices for prescription-based painkillers and other pharmaceuticals. In fact, the American Association of Retired Persons has found that prescription drug prices have shot up far higher than the inflation rate.

Frustrated, angered and even left feeling hopeless due to this critical distribution system, many people repeat this commonly used observation—"Only in America do drugstores make the sick walk all the way to the back of the store to get their prescriptions,

physical injuries, or perhaps even from the ravages of disease such as cancer.

In many cases of neuropathic pain, the patient describes feeling hurt in an area of the body other than where the wound or disease occurred. This sometimes happens because specific or widespread sections of the overall nervous system have been severely damaged. Generally, physicians list neuropathic pain into two categories. They are:

- **Superficial Somatic:** Sometimes described as "deep pain" or deep somatic pain, these occur when nociceptors transmit sensations of poorly localized, dull or aching pains from muscles, ligaments, bones, tendons, blood vessels and other areas.

- **Visceral Pain:** These unwelcome sensations emanate from the organs, but physicians often have difficulty locating a specific site. Patients sometimes describe these sensations as "pins and needles," or stabbing, burning, electrical or tingling.

Meantime, neuropathic pain is transmitted to the brain via either of two sections of the nervous system. One involves the central nervous system originating from the spinal cord and brain. And the other encompasses the peripheral nervous system, emanating from areas of the body unprotected by the blood-brain barrier, skull, or spine. The blood-brain barrier is an area separate from the central nervous system.

Consider Pain as a Symptom Rather Than a Condition

For the most part, pain emerges only as a symptom of one or more medical conditions. As unbelievable as this might sound, pain is not the underlying problem or root cause of an original debilitating medical condition. Instead, this sensation occurs as a result of a specific biological problem such as a disease, heart attack a wound, or a physical or chemical injury.

Except for instances where the nervous system or areas of the brain are damaged, the instances where a person naturally fails to feel pain include:

- **Unconsciousness:** A patient is rendered unconscious, to the point where he or she fails to realize that pain is occurring. Sometimes comas occur naturally as the body's way of blocking pain, so that the organs can heal. For this reason, especially for certain cases involving severe injury, physicians sometimes intentionally induce comas in order to provide for a pain-free period for the body's natural restoration and healing processes to work.

- **Death:** Some or all of a particular appendage, limb or organ dies along with any sections of the nervous system within that area. Heart attacks usually result in the death of certain sections of that organ, and gangrene can kill large or small areas of the body. Frostbite also can kill peripheral areas of the body, while leaving other areas relatively healthy or intact.

With all these considerations in mind, after initially taking short-term measures to relieve pain upon seeing a new patient for the first time, many physicians immediately seek to locate and cure the underlying or primary condition that causes the discomfort.

"This is only going to hurt a little," some medical professionals such as dental assistant tell patients, immediately before rendering shots containing pain-blocking substances. Sometimes, such statements are a "lie," because these injections may create extreme discomfort that soon dissipates when the local anesthetic takes effect.

Severe Pain Can Contribute to Shock That Results in Death

Although pain is a symptom rather than an underlying medical condition, the sensation can play a potential role in severe circulatory failure—potentially resulting in imminent or sudden death.

Along with the potentially fatal loss of blood or the loss of vital organs, people who suffer from traumatic injuries such as car wrecks or who battle wounds face the possibility of circulatory shock—commonly known as "shock"—a life threatening condition that refers to a blood pressure less than 80.

In some of these critical medical events, extreme pain ravages individuals who remain partially or fully conscious. Amid or shortly following such events, the sudden elimination of pain via the use of narcotics such as morphine can help play a significant role in enabling medical professionals or battlefield medics to stabilize a patient's overall medical condition. This sometimes opens a pathway for additional treatments and, hopefully, eventual recovery.

Physicians have chronicled many types of circulatory shock, almost all of them potentially fatal. These range from septic shock that involves the loss of blood circulation from bacterial infection to vital organs and to hypovolaemic shock that occurs due to extreme blood loss and falling blood pressure.

Circulatory shock can lead to various life-ending events or conditions, such as cardiac arrest where the heart stops and hypoxemia where arterial blood fails to receive a necessary and essential supply of oxygen.

Ignoring Pain Can Result in Death

Early detection, in many cases thanks to the initial onset of pain, can lead to reversal of serious medical conditions, possibly resulting in a return to good health. Statistics provided by a wide variety of health organizations indicate the definite benefits of early detection of diseases ranging from heart problems to cancer.

According to documentation provided by the American Cancer Society, "regular use of some established screening tests can prevent the development of cancer through identification and removal or treatment of pre-malignant abnormalities. Screening tests can also improve survival and decrease mortality by deleting cancer at an early stage when treatment is more effective." The society has published its annual Cancer Prevention and Early Detection Facts and Figures since 1992.

For people suffering from chest pains or severe aches in the jaw, neck, shoulders, back or arms—particularly on the body's left side—the American Heart Association recommends getting immediate medical attention. Necessary or recommended tests during—or immediately after such episodes—include documentation of a complete medical history, a complete physical examination, an electrocardiogram and blood tests.

Besides potential heart or cancer problems, a wide range of other possible diseases that pain can signal range from the onset of arthritis, cholera, muscular ailments, malaria, the flu, lung disease, circulatory problems, Lyme disease, and many others. In many instances some of these afflictions are first noticed via the onset of pain, including numerous afflictions that can emerge as debilitating or fatal unless detected early.

Common sense dictates that all of us should heed the early warning signs of pain, rather than risk having physicians discover what we consider the worst possible outcomes. As the widely acclaimed genius Albert Einstein once proclaimed: "God does not play dice."

Pain Can Sometimes Serve as a Blessing

No matter how much we try to think otherwise, pain can emerge as a wonderful blessing. Yes, physical pain can warn us when something has gone terribly wrong with our bodies, potentially notifying us to take necessary and decisive medical action. Emotional agony and heartache also can serve as integral signals of severe internal distress.

People who suffer from chronic or unexpected pain should:

- **Notify:** Visit a physician, medical professional or health care facility as soon as possible.

- **Vigilant:** Adhere to recommended or prescribed treatments without getting off track.

- **Follow-Up:** Schedule and keep subsequent medical appointments to track the progress of disease or injury in order to implement or modify treatments to get the best pain-relieving results.

According to many news reports, women are far more likely to get regular medical check-ups in response to pain. Some medical professionals and analysts believe this occurs because men are less likely than women to want to discuss or share personal issues involving stress, emotions and depression—known potential pain triggers. The only major exception, at least by some accounts, entails matters of sexual dysfunction, instances where men often eagerly seek medical help and advice.

An age-old saying dictates that "trouble is part of your life and if you don't share it, you don't give the person who loves you a chance to love you enough." When matters of physical pain become involved, we all should love ourselves enough to seek professional help, particularly as soon as we begin suffering unexpected physical distress.

Pain Leads to Other Severe Conditions

Countless people worldwide have chosen to commit suicide

because they could no longer endure pain that medications failed to relieve. Besides suicide, chronic and debilitating physical pain often leads to a wide variety of extremely severe mental and physical conditions. Key among these is chronic depression, a mental disorder called by a wide variety of names. People suffering from severe physical pain sometimes experience some of the worst symptoms or attributes of chronic depression.

Often suffering so much physical pain that they become disabled, those experiencing chronic depression sometimes lose their sense of self worth. A common complaint involves an inability to seek or experience pleasure.

When this occurs, virtually everything in a person's lifestyle is impacted. Chronic depression adversely impacts family life, the ability to effectively interact with other individuals, and the ability to perform or achieve basic goals at school or at work.

Despite such observations, there is no denying that chronic depression is an extremely serious condition that can lead to a variety of negative physical conditions. Such situations often adversely impact all vital aspects of generally good health, ranging from sleeping and eating habits to the lack of a healthy sex life.

Exacerbating matters, certain pharmaceuticals that are administered in hopes of alleviating or masking the effects of physical pain sometimes lead to mood disorders. Also compounding the problem, these difficulties can potentially worsen to the point that the immune system weakens, leading to or increasing the probability of severe infections.

Faced with such extreme potential outcomes, patients and physicians find themselves challenged by the need to face physical pain and its causes head-on. Only through such direct efforts can effective results occur. The ultimate goal always remains the total elimination or the masking of physical pain, thereby opening up a pathway toward potential happiness or at least the resumption of average, common lifestyles.

"To enjoy good health, to bring true happiness to one's family, to bring peace to all, one must first discipline and control one's own mind," said the Buddha, a spiritual teacher and the founder of Buddhism in about the fifth century before Christ. "If a man can control his mind, he can find the way to enlightenment, and all wisdom and virtue will naturally come to him."

Chapter 2

Real or Imagined, Pain Takes Many Forms

The Mysteries of Phantom Pain

Since at least the 1500s, physicians have heard patients complain of perceived pain in areas where limbs have been severed or extremities removed. The lay public often refers to such instances as "phantom limb pain."

Besides phantom limb sensations, medical professionals from many cultures have documented cases where patients also describe "phantom limb sensations." These people get sensations that all or portions of their missing limbs remain attached to their bodies.

American neurologist Silas Weir Mitchell chronicled the existence of phantom limbs in 1871, writing that "thousands of spirit limbs were haunting as many good soldiers, (and) every now and then tormenting them." Some startled or mystified patients insisted that the existence of their missing but still-felt limbs seemed real to them, feeling as if having the same mass and weight as any remaining appendages.

I do believe in ghosts," said Devon Joseph Werkheiser, an American actor and writer. "Freaky things will happen, and I'm like, 'the wind didn't do that. Some spirit did.'" Although the phenomenon of phantom pain and phantom limbs might seem otherworldly, medical professionals insist they have developed logical and conclusive findings that show these attributes exist—at least in the minds of certain patients.

Judging by some accounts, physicians have yet to develop a universally accepted theory on how and why these sensations occur. In any case, the prevalence of and similarities among such cases persist. The phenomena also sometimes involve people who have only portions of certain limbs due to birth defects.

Some physicians believe these varying sensations develop within the peripheral, spinal or central nervous system areas. Adding to the mystery, researchers also have insisted that the thalamus, the cortex and the body's limbic system of various structures and processes within the brain can essentially make the patient believe that a missing limb still exists.

In many of these cases physicians sometimes find themselves faced with the need to eliminate their patients' sensations of pain in limbs that no longer exist. Some doctors have gone so far as to prescribe pain-reducing medications, or even antidepressants or drugs used to control epileptic seizures. These efforts occasionally have generated some success.

Desperate for effective relief, some patients suffering from persistent phantom limb pain have undergone what physicians call specialized "mirror box" treatments. A percentage of these patients perceive pain in phantom limbs that remain clinched, at least from the perceptions of their own minds. But since the limbs do not exist, the patients are unable to naturally unclench muscles of the missing limbs—a process that people with all their appendages often use to eliminate cramps or muscular discomfort.

Some researchers think that the brain gradually starts believing that the missing limb remains intact. All along, however, the brain also incorrectly senses on occasion that the phantom appendage fails to send messages due to apparent paralysis. To correct this problem, some medical professionals strive to give the brain visual feedback via the "mirror box" process, thereby creating an impression that the limb has moved.

Medical professions occasionally use mirrors in order to develop this desired visual impression, thereby creating an image that the missing limb still exists. Upon seeing this image live in a mirror, the patient is instructed to send motor or mental orders to the missing limb and to the remaining opposite limb to make symmetric or similar movements. The objective is to make the brain believe that the missing limb has actually moved, while no longer paralyzed.

In a sense, it would seem that medical professionals need to emulate the role of magicians, to switch the brain into a recovery mode via the use of visual trickery or at least creating false illusions.

"In the many years that I have been before the public, my secret methods have been steadily shielded," said Harry Houdini, an American magician and stunt performer. The magic secrets "have been shielded by the strict integrity of my assistants, most of whom have been with me for years."

Unlike such entertainers, medical professionals can and should continue to share their various successes in order to develop the most effective treatment methods.

The Lack of Pain Adds to the Mystery

As if the basic physical properties involving physical pain weren't already enough to amaze and confound researchers, there also are rare cases of people who fail to feel any such sensations whatsoever.

Referred to by physicians as "congenital insensitivity to pain" or "congenital analgesia," an extremely small percentage of people are born with an inability to suffer physical pain. Researchers also have concluded that some instances of congenital insensitivity to pain might be hereditary, passed from parents to their children. Progressive illnesses such as Hansen's Disease—commonly known as "leprosy"—can progressively destroy the nerves. Thereafter, scientists fear, the parents could possibly pass the illness to their offspring.

While serving as a primary and necessary essence of life, physical pain fails us when such sensations disappear and thereby become unable to do their job of signaling problems. Paradoxically, the permanent lack of such sensations becomes just as tragic as feeling physical pain. Each occurrence expresses a great potential problem. They are:

- **Feeling Pain:** The sensations of too much physical pain can gradually or suddenly bring about painful emotional situations as well, sometimes robbing people of the will to live or stealing away any hope of recovery.

- **Lacking Any Pain**: Countless diseases or potential injuries might erupt while the individual and his necessary immune system response mode fail in duties to react to illness and wounds. This, in turn, might prevent the nerves from sending to the brain critical information about pain in order for the person to generate adequate or necessary responses for healing. Thus, the complete and permanent lack of pain persists.

In 2005, *People* magazine reported the compelling story of Ashlyn Blocker, who at age 5 suffered from congenital insensitivity to pain. Among the child's various pain-inducing behaviors reported by the magazine:

- **Head:** Slammed her head against the walls, shrugging at the site of blood on her face.

   Hand: Left her hand in the muffler of a gas-powered mower.

- **Fingers:** Put her fingers into a door frame, before the device crushed them.

- **Ants**: Failed to notice when hundreds of ants started biting her, instead telling relatives that she couldn't get the dirt off her skin.

- **Mouth:** Badly bit her own lips, cheeks, and tongue, "causing so much damage that she began knocking out her front teeth."

"She looks like a little boxer," her mother told the magazine. "We don't want Ashlyn to live in a bubble. We've learned what to worry about and what not to worry about, and we give her space."

Her family and medical professionals were striving to teach her how to detect signs of potential infections such as appendicitis. Following this extensive education process, Ashlyn learned to find her mother whenever she saw blood, and to ask if food was cool enough to eat.

"She's got the best laugh in the world," Tara said, adding that "I would give anything, absolutely anything, for Ashlyn to feel pain."

Psychosomatic Situations Complicate the Field of Pain

Complicating the overall study, diagnosis and treatment of standard pain, many people also suffer from what physicians refer to as "psychosomatic behavior." This condition involves bodily symptoms caused by a mental or emotional disturbance.

In many cases involving psychosomatic symptoms of pain, physicians often cite emotional or physical stress as a primary instigating factor. Intertwining this mix, chronic physical stress also can lead to general or "actual" illness.

Both lay people and medical professionals need to remain cognizant that an individual sometimes suffers stress in situations where he or she feels a complete or near-total lack of ability to control unpleasant events. Major potential stressors could include everything from an inability to generate a sufficient income to worries about a lover's potential infidelity or earning adequate grades in school.

Many people tend to place unwarranted blame on those who experience psychosomatic medical conditions. Anyone who would call such a patient "nuts" or "loony" should seriously consider withholding such thoughts. After all, as a result of their perceived conditions, psychosomatics sometimes suffer emotionally, spiritually and financially while also experiencing potentially debilitating physical symptoms.

Some of the world's most respected behavioral experts still insist on placing blame on psychosomatics for bringing about their own medical conditions. As a result, this complex and often poorly understood issue will likely remain a hot topic, even as new and much-wanted medical advances gradually evolve.

"Win-lose people bury a lot of feelings. And unexpressed feelings come forth later in uglier ways," said Stephen R. Covey, author of the bestseller "The Seven Habits of Highly Effective People." "Psychosomatic illnesses often are the reincarnation of cumulative resentment, deep disappointment and disillusionment repressed by the win-lose mentality."

Whether or not they agree with such assessments physicians need to treat such conditions with just as much care and concern as any other serious medical condition.

Within the extensive overall practice of behavioral medicine, the detection and effective treatment of psychosomatic behavior can depend on variations of a wide range of specialties. These can include—but are not necessarily limited to—everything from psychiatry, physiology, and allergies to dermatology, and many more areas of medicine.

Psychosomatics often complain of either specific or vague pains, some described as severe or mild. After at least a short time in practice, just about every new doctor has heard a patient describe a small or vast array of perceived physical complaints that lack any underlying standard medical basis.

More than merely a figment of the psychosomatic patient's imagination, these perceived ailments including the perceptions of pain are very "real" in their minds. In fact, the force of the mind is so powerful that some psychosomatics experience or express observable symptoms such as rashes, convulsions or body temperature changes.

"You have power over your mind, not outside events," said Marcus Aurelius, a Roman emperor in the second century after Christ. "Realize this, and you will find strength."

Many physicians and medical professionals focus on the use of positive thinking or even what some lay people refer to as "mind over matter." This is not to imply in any way whatsoever that physicians strive to employ treatments that delve into the paranormal. Instead, many treatment experts emphasize the spiritual realm of the personal belief system generated within the mind, which some people believe holds just as much great power as the body.

Psychosomatic Medicine Has a Vibrant, Important History

Historians tell us that physicians have known about psychosomatics since at least the 10th Century, when two psychologists and physicians first noted these conditions during the medieval Islamic period. Through their studies, research and medical practices, Ahmed ibn Sahl al-Balkhi and Haly Abbas determined that the psychology and physiology of a patient can impact each other.

These physicians noted correlations between people who are both mentally and physically ill, and those who are healthy. Then, during the 11th Century, a famed Persian physician and philosopher known today by the single name "Avicenna," recognized and described the significant impact that emotions can play on our bodies.

Significant advances occurred in the study and identification of psychosomatics throughout the 20th Century, particularly beginning in the early 1970s when many physicians started using the biosemiotic theory as a basis for such medicine. A German, Thure von Uexküll, a scholar of psychosomatic medicine, and his colleagues, developed the biosemiotic theory that attempts to:

● **Integrate**: Melding the conclusions researchers have

made in scientific biology and "semiotics," a term used to describe the studies of the symbols and signs from various cultures. In the view of John Locke, the 17th Century English philosopher, semiotics can relate to everything from words, to the nature of things, and their relationships with each other. In the 19th Century, American scientist, philosopher and mathematician Charles Sanders Peirce defined semiotics as signs used by "intelligence capable of learning by experience."

- **Interpretation:** This is the process where people assign meaning to the various signs, symbols and messages, often via verbal messages or by sight. Without necessarily knowing this is being done, a person sometimes uses his perceptions of logic or mathematical data to interpret information that arrives in the forms of signs or symbols.

- **Paradigmatic shift:** The blending of scientific biology and semiotics causes a "paradigmatic shift," a term used to describe changes in previously accepted basics that involve the theory of science.

This complex integration and interaction of the basic science of biology with the system of signs or messages can effect a person's perception of life.

Jakob Johann von Uexküll, a Baltic German biologist in the late 1800s and early 1900s, used the "unwelt" theory that people and other animals can generate or interpret different meanings from certain signs or communications—although they share a similar environment. This "unwelt" concept also is often considered to play a significant role in the approach that today's physicians, psychiatrists and medical professionals take when dealing with the psychosomatic phenomenon.

Physicians report that people experiencing psychosomatic medical conditions often suffer from one or more physical diseases, stemming from life's everyday stresses. Psychiatry has made recent advances in determining which mental factors—if any— were the likely cause of a specific individual's psychosomatic-related medical problem.

The wide array of documented medical conditions include Irritable Bowel Syndrome, chronic fatigue syndrome, peptic ulcers, lower back pain, bacterial infections, and high blood pressure. Some of these maladies can emerge as serious and sometimes life-threatening medical conditions.

All along, scientists and medical professions stress the importance of avoiding any use of the incorrect term "psychosomatic illness," when referring to certain types of mental illnesses or "somatoform disorders." Individuals experiencing the mental illness of somatoform disorders sometimes exhibit physical symptoms similar to those conditions experienced by people who have been in accidents or who have certain illnesses.
In summary, the basic differences between these overall conditions

- **Somatoform disorders:** This is a disorder that can result from various mental factors. Such patients often become unnecessarily worried or stressed when physicians are unable to diagnose a specific cause, a determination necessary to describe a pain or an ailment.

- **Psychosomatic medicine:** This is a field of medicine that involves various medical specialties, hinged largely on the bodily processes and on the health of people. Personal behaviors, social conditions and psychology are among factors that play key roles. As a subspecialty of psychiatry and neurology, this condition also can sometimes benefit from positive thinking or what physicians sometimes call "the power of suggestion."

Ultimately, as with any serious medical condition, patients should never attempt to diagnose themselves, particularly in matters that involve real or perceived pain. Only a certified and licensed medical professional can make an accurate diagnosis, before recommending and implementing treatments or prescriptions.

Worsening matters from the perspective of patients, the various conditions involving psychosomatic medicine and somatoform disorders can result in what lay people and even physicians sometimes refer to as a "pain disorder." Such conditions can become so severe that a patient sometimes becomes disabled, preventing him or her from common everyday activities.

As with most severe medical conditions, those suffering from intense pain should visit a physician or medical professional as soon as possible. Early diagnosis and treatment could possibly go a long way toward stopping or preventing the progression of symptoms. According to some researchers, the onset of any pain disorder can hit both genders at any age.

Taking on a so-called "life of its own," some instances of pain disorder reportedly stem from an actual injury or illness. Thereafter, following the point when the underlying or primary medical condition is otherwise "cured," the patient continues to perceive severe pain or discomfort—when in fact there is no underlying medical basis for such symptoms. Indeed, the accurate diagnosis of "real" or "perceived" pain is an extremely complex and integral process that sometimes involves extensive medical testing over an extended period of time

Chapter 3

Many Pain Treatments
Have Deep Roots

Since the beginning of recorded history humans have created diverse belief systems, remedies, technologies and medical systems with the primary goal of relieving pain. Many cultures attributed physical pains, severe illness and mental stresses on the presumed or supposed "will of the gods," or attributed painful conditions to everything from witchcraft to the positioning of stars for the emergence of certain painful conditions. Such prevalent beliefs in such systems gradually faded for the most part thanks to the eventual advent and emergence of modern science.

Anthropologists and sociologists tell us that many pre-historic cultures from such diverse regions as North America to the Congo almost always looked to a single, central figure for advice or to take action in the hoped-for healing process. To the North American tribes, these individuals were often hailed as the "medicine man." To Eskimos and Siberians, such individuals were "shamans," while some jungle-based cultures such as those in the Congo referred to these individuals as "witch doctors."

Tribes or clans looked to one individual to handle the essential role of eliminating pain or curing illness; other societies or cultures sought the help of a group of healers formed within secret societies. Certain individuals were allowed into these positions or groups only after demonstrating that they had experienced persistent dreams about possible remedies or reasons for illness.

Perhaps these overall ancient, antiquated requirements mirror much of today's mainstream allopathic medical practices, including methods that sometimes are considered mandatory although the techniques are ineffective. A key example might be the excessive or unnecessary employment of extreme levels of chemotherapies, even in instances where standard science and historic results indicate such treatments provide little or no effective results.

Early Cultures Began Using Plants and Herbs

Many early cultures, particularly in North America, gradually began using specific plants and herbs to treat ailments or perceived problems that included sore throats, constipation, sleeplessness, and pain relievers. Many of these early remedies became the basis for herbs and human-produced drugs widely prescribed by modern medical professionals. Among the early medical successes of ancient peoples:

- **Herbs and minerals:** Developed or identified herbs or other substances, deemed effective in the treatments of specific types of medical complaints.

- **Trial and error:** At least partly mirroring modern scientists efforts to undergo rigorous testing in the research and development process, pre-historic cultures pinpointed which substances worked and which failed at addressing specific ailments.

- **Long-term efforts:** Early cultures realized that many of the worst diseases or illnesses only hit an individual once—never returning again after immunity developed. For this reason, some people within specific pre-historic cultures apparently strived to suffer from mild cases of specific illnesses in order to prevent becoming extremely sick in the future.

Many if not most of these early efforts lacked a rock-solid, scientific basis. For the most part, early medicine men were merely embracing or practicing the spiritual belief systems and traditions passed from generation to generation within their own cultures.

It remains clear that lots of people suffering from severe pains thousands of years ago probably demanded, pleaded for or sought the types of remedies that many of us take for granted today. Some researchers have even argued or at least suggested that pre-historic people even employed healing clays—or "medicinal clays"—for certain healing or medicinal qualities, mimicking remedies used by certain wild animals.

Anthropologists have reported finding signs of widespread use of medicinal clays among various ancient indigenous cultures including Mesopotamia. Researchers believe people externally applied these materials to the skin during certain activities, such as bathing at health spas or taking mud baths.

At least some aspects of these early pre-historic or ancient-period traditions continue even today, particularly within certain realms of alternative medicine. For the most part, such treatments or applications are not recognized by practitioners of today's "standard, mainstream medicine" as having medically viable or therapeutic qualities.

Scientists and practitioners of homeopathic medicine sometimes refer to the use of clays for medicinal purposes as "geophagy." Even the famous ancient Greek physician and philosopher Galen noticed that certain wild animals including reptiles, birds and mammals sometime use clay to treat their illnesses or injuries.

While many mainstream physicians argue otherwise, numerous homeopaths and practitioners of alternative medicine insist that some medicinal clays possess indisputable antibacterial qualities, making these materials effective in the treatment of surface pains.

According to an article in the *Journal of Antimicroborial Chemotherapy*, certain iron-rich clays have been effective in killing some bacteria within test tubes. And, a 2008 article entitled "Healing Clays," stated that at least 20 of these bentonite-type materials showed promising results in fighting the "super-bug" bacterium MRSA—scientifically called "Methicillin-resistant Staphylococcus aureus."

As controversy continues to erupt as to the effectiveness of medicinal clays first used thousands of years ago, therapeutic mud baths remain increasingly popular within many cultures. And some mainstream medical facilities have experimented with the use of such substances at least in part for the treatment of war wounds. A 2008 article in *Wired* noted that chemists had infused gauze with nano-particles of clay, drastically improving the ability to curtail blood loss.

These are just a few examples of why scientists and physicians determined to whip the ravages of pain should continue researching and possibly implementing potential medical treatments first used long ago by ancient people.

Serious Pain Treatments Emerged 4,000 Years Ago

Concerted efforts to address pain and related ailments began about 2,000 years before Christ in the Egyptian, Mesopotamian and Babylonian cultures, according to various archeological reports and scientific documents. For the most part many medical advances and strategies in these regions avoided mysticism or citing the gods as reasons for painful ailments, but instead focused on potential scientific causes.

Particularly in the early Babylonian culture, physicians gradually began the process of diagnosing specific illnesses. These early doctors conducted physical examinations before stating the prognosis or projected outcomes of specific individual patients. Along with the advent of issuing prescriptions, all these basic steps gradually emerged worldwide as the foundations and basic standards for today's general pain-fighting medical practices.

According to various quotations from the Bible's early sections, around 1,000 years before Christ the Hebrews realized the vital interaction between cleanliness and the prospects for good, pain-free health. Those early findings and advances in cultural changes established the necessary foundation for the ongoing need to keep materials free of germs and away from potentially harmful bacteria to lessen the probability of infections.

That age-old saying that "cleanliness is next to godliness," still holds true more than ever before—especially in matters involving the effective elimination, prevention and eradication of pain or the primary medical conditions that ignite such sensations.

"Keep your spirits up and your physical body as clean as possible," I tell many of my patients today. Besides good nutrition, a steady exercise regimen and adequate periods for sleep, keeping the body's surface free of potential infectious-causing viruses can go a long way in helping you to achieve and to maintain overall good, pain-free health.

While the early foundations of today's mainstream standard medical practice evolved in Europe and the Middle East, early precursors of modern alternative treatments came about in vastly different regions of the world such as China. Within the Chinese culture, the prescribing of herbs and various natural plant-based substances for pain and illness is considered "mainstream." But for many people in the Western culture, particularly in the United States, such treatments are viewed as "alternative." Most such pain-fighting efforts that evolved in the Chinese culture, such as herbs and acupuncture, remain unrecognized by standard allopathic physicians in the U.S., where giant for-profit pharmaceutical companies rule the marketplace.

The basic culture of the USA ignores and even shuns the

remarkable treatments first developed in China and other non-European countries thousands of years ago.

Perhaps this aspect—the occasional use of vital, pain-killing or health-enhancing herbs through my medical practice—angers or upsets some standard medical practitioners. In a sense, from their view, my treatment methods have rocked the proverbial apple cart. Is it possible that mainstream physicians feel threatened, as people from all over the world flock to my medical clinic in the Western United States?

Remember that while striving to fight and eliminate the pain and other ailments that my patients experience, as an integrative practitioner of medicine I sometimes use or prescribe herbal treatments or natural pain remedies that have proven effective for thousands of years within other cultures of the world.

Early Chinese Medicines Can Help Fight Pain

Although many of today's mainstream American medical professionals might tell you otherwise, some of the various herbs, acupuncture methods and massages developed in early China can play a significant role in fighting pain.

Some critics argue that Chinese-based treatments ignore standard and acceptable scientific medical criteria. Perhaps such criticism stems at least in part from the fact that traditional Chinese medicine views the interconnection among the body's various organs at least partly on the basis of certain metaphysical principles. This emerges as a sharp contrast from mainstream medicines in our Western culture, where science-based medicine prevails—hinged largely on specific research involving specific bodily functions.

By contrast, since emerging thousands of years ago, basic medical practices embraced by the Chinese culture blame illness on an imbalance among the body's various sections and functional organs.

As you might imagine, some mainstream traditional doctors in our Western culture whine like little babies when they see that growing numbers of patients worldwide agree with my analysis in this regard. To these upset doctors, I have to say that "why should we ignore and refuse to recognize effective treatments that a vast majority of the world's people use and fully accept? And, just because an overall standard allopathic treatment method is developed in the United States—hooked largely to big pharmaceutical companies—why should those systems be considered better in every instance, relegated as the only viable options?"

Generally, the practitioners of Chinese medicines strive to use everything from herbs and minerals to animal products and acupuncture in treating particular inter-related organ systems. Many of the harshest critics are quick to say that such treatments lack any verifiable and quantifiable scientific basis, while producing questionable results.

Such critics undoubtedly cringe at video presentations on my Web site, DrForsythe.com. These heart-felt, compelling and magnetic proclamations come from steadily growing numbers of my patients from around the world. Some of these emotional statements feature patients who had once lost hope for physical improvements before my treatments left them pain-free or at least feeling less pain and suffering.

Other Ancient Cultures Contributed to Alternative Medicines

As controversy continues to erupt about the effectiveness of homeopathic medicine, we need to remain mindful that a wide variety of other cultures besides the Chinese also made significant contributions to today's alternative treatment systems.

The various cultures, nations and continents where natural plant-based remedies evolved during the past 2,000 years include the Germanic region, the vast areas of Central America and South America and across much of Africa as well. Through trial and error, cultures that followed the pre-historic era found or rediscovered essential plants and minerals that are often prescribed today by homeopaths for pain treatments.

Through the Middle Ages between the fifth century after Christ and the 1400s, regions including the weakening Western Roman and Eastern Roman empires strived to identify and develop more effective treatments for various painful and sometimes fatal illnesses. Historians tell us that during this period as a crossroads between the east and the west Persia served as an integral site during the developments of ancient Indian and Greek medicines.

As the Islamic civilization grew and prospered, Arab physicians played central roles in developing new and essential medical systems. These ranged from surgeries to pharmacies and the development of various pharmaceutical products, including some for the treatment of pain.

Meantime, during the same 1,000-year span, as the authority of the former Roman Empire disintegrated, Christian-based societies and cultures began independently developing, embracing or formalizing the medical infrastructure. While hospitals started emerging, some medical professionals began to drop the ancient teachings of the Romans and Greeks on how to treat pain— and instead commenced the development of new and unique treatments, often based on their own observations.

Rapid and essential advancements followed through the Renaissance, from the 14th through the 17th centuries, when a cultural movement embraced the development of the arts and the sciences throughout most of Europe. At an increasingly rapid pace during this period, physicians and scientists began examining the bodies of living people, dissected cadavers and launched a vast array of experiments.

Essentially, all this was done in large part in an effort to determine the causes of the body's various physical pains, how those signals were identified, transmitted to and interpreted by the brain, and possible ways of treating or eliminating such sensations.

Chapter 4

Wars Advanced
Our Understnding of Pain

Whether we like to admit this or not, throughout history, especially during the last 300 years, the world's bloodiest wars played a pivotal role in enabling physicians to learn more about the phenomena of pain and to develop more effective treatments.

"Doctors will have more lives to answer for in the next world than even we generals," said Napoleon Bonaparte, the French emperor and military leader. Particularly from the Renaissance through the present day, as the weapons employed in wars became increasingly sophisticated and battle zones stretched for thousands of miles, physicians were forced to treat on a massive scale everything from wounds to extreme hunger and diseases such as dysentery.

Many wars throughout history have ravaged and decimated vast cultures. But the intensity, number and ferocity of such conflicts intensified in the 1700s. The Great Northern War stretching from 1700 to 1721 started this era of seemingly non-stop death and destruction involving 13 countries or empires from Great Britain to the Ottoman Empire. This marked just the start of the horrors that were to plague that era; historians tell us that at least 70 wars erupted worldwide during the 1700s, including the American Revolutionary War.

Lacking the fast-paced medical technology prevalent on today's battlefields, during those clashes tens of thousands—and collectively perhaps millions—of soldiers suffered horrifically painful wounds. Many of them were left mortally wounded on battlefields, stricken by wretched and hellish pains. Lots of these victims spent their final minutes, hours or even days, wailing for help or relief from pain that never subsided until unconsciousness and eventual death, which many of them apparently welcomed after intense suffering.

Physicians from the Union and Confederate armies made tremendous gains during the American Civil War, during which an estimated 260,000 soldiers died and perhaps tens of thousands suffered the loss of limbs. Huge casualty totals in many bloody battles forced physicians to devise methods of quickly alleviating extreme pain, enabling doctors or medical crews to administer life-saving battlefield amputations. Some basic techniques these physicians devised emerged as the forefront of primary pain-fighting strategies employed today in both war and peacetime environments.

Historians tell us that wars elsewhere before this great American confrontation mostly featured relatively small armies, primarily due to the logistical challenges of amassing troops, plus the difficulties of generating efficient supply lines. And, prior to the Civil War, notoriously inaccurate musket fire kept casualties to a minimum.

Those trends took a sharp reversal during the American confrontation as trains, supply lines and new telegraph systems increased efficiency. Adding to the misery, the advent of mass-produced canned foods and vastly more efficient Minié ball weaponry enabled massive numbers of troops to essentially become efficient killing machines in high numbers in confined areas.

Within months after the war erupted, the Union Army began requiring that each regiment recruit at least one surgeon and one assistant surgeon. When mobile medical transportation systems proved inefficient as thousands of soldiers died, the military developed an all-new ambulance corps in order to accelerate transportation of the pain-stricken, wounded soldiers to hospitals. Although relatively crude by today's standards, these systems emerged as to the early precursors to today's modern ambulance systems. Even then doctors realized the urgency of getting patients treatment as soon as possible in order to treat pain, injury, illness and hemorrhaging.

Physical and Emotional Pains Became a Top Priority

The steadily increasing magnitude and intensity of the war forced the Union to upgrade transportation, hospitals, nursing crews and in-the-field educational procedures by early 1863. Meantime, the Confederates' medical core was organized much faster but it lacked the non-stop supply of vital and essential pain-killers and surgeons available in the north.

On both sides, for the first time in the history of war soldiers and their industrial supporters strived to amass extensive non-stop quantities of alcohol and the organic compound of chloroform in an effort to alleviate pains suffered by the continually swelling numbers of severely wounded.

Much of the time while undergoing amputations, the patients remained at least somewhat awake while never realizing much of the resulting pain, at least according to some published accounts. From the standpoint of today's physicians such as me, these developments—although relatively crude and non-sophisticated in nature—marked a significant development in the treatment of sudden, intense and debilitating pain.

Stewart Brand, an American writer best known as editor of the *Whole Earth Catalogue*, has been quoted as saying that "Once a new technology rolls over you, if you're not part of the steamroller, you're part of the road." Sure enough, historians tell us that these new or upgraded pain-killing methods on a massive scale forced battlefield physicians to intensify and continually improve their pain fighting methods.

In the form of a sweet-smelling liquid, the chloroform soon gained a well-deserved reputation as extremely dangerous. Derived primarily from naturally occurring ocean-based substances such as seaweed, chloroform started gaining popularity as an anesthetic in 1847, just 14 years before the Civil War erupted.

Chloroform's earliest use as an anesthetic emerged when a Scottish physician, James Young Simpson, began administering the substance to women undergoing childbirth. The popularity of using this substance soon spread as increasing numbers of physicians realized chloroform's ability to suppress the central nervous system, the body's system of communicating pain signals from the site of a wound to the brain.

By the time the Civil War began some U.S. surgeons and general physicians had already started using chloroform. The war quickly brought chloroform to the forefront as the general public began perceiving the substance to be a crucial tool in fighting or warding off pain, especially during amputations or extensive surgeries.

The widespread popularity of chloroform took a sharp downswing, especially during the initial decades after the war. Physicians and their patients gradually began to realize and acknowledge chloroform's toxicity, which sometimes caused what some people hailed as "sudden sniffer's death," commonly known today as sudden cardiac arrhythmia.

Through much of the mid-1800s chloroform emerged as a preferred anesthetic, temporarily exceeding the popularity of ether. But ether re-emerged as a predominant favorite by the early 20th Century as physicians began avoiding the use of chloroform.

The Ether Pain Killer Swelled in Popularity

From the 1200s through the 1500s, scientists, researchers and physicians began to realize and appreciate the pain-killing attributes of ether, a colorless and highly flammable liquid created when distilling a mixture of sulfuric acid and ethanol. During that period, doctors began to recognize ether's indisputable qualities as an "analgesic," the term used in designating any specific drug as a painkiller.

In the 1840s, the physician Crawford Williamson Long demonstrated in private sessions the use of ether as a general anesthetic. Soon afterward, in Boston, William T.G. Morton gave a public demonstration of the use of ether as a general anesthetic.

Even today, at least judging by some news accounts, ether hails as a preferred choice as a general anesthetic in some developing nations where the substance remains readily available thanks to its relatively low cost when compared to the most popular drugs in its class. However, like many other powerful pharmaceutical products that target pain, ether became a "recreational drug" that some people abused because of its impact on the central nervous system.

An ancient Chinese proverb proclaims that "it is easy to get a thousand prescriptions, but hard to get one single remedy." Indeed, especially during the late 1800s, people began devising, producing or distributing various types of analgesics at a rapidly increasing rate, even some substances that had been known for thousands of years but that had received little overall publicity until then. As a result, society began to recognize and even ban or discourage some substances due to their negative side effects.

Some greedy companies and individual consumers eager to profit from or abuse painkillers devised crafty methods of distributing and consuming such substances. Certain cough drops during this period contained both ether and alcohol. Many of the most ardent consumers of these products reportedly were women, perhaps because adult females were often banned or discouraged from attending social events where men enjoyed drinking alcohol.

In John Irving's novel, *The Cider House Rules*, which later became a 1999 Academy Award-winning movie by the same name, the character Dr. Wilbur Larch portrayed by Michael Caine in the film, succumbs to an addiction to ether consumption. The fictional doctor dies at the beginning of the 20th Century at an orphanage. This award-winning book and film epitomized the social views of the early 20th Century, when some emerging analgesics became vilified and shunned almost as quickly as they had surged in popularity.

Major Strides Against Pain Developed
in Iraq and Afghanistan Wars

The concept and process of pain management has accelerated thanks to major advances developed by U.S. military medical personnel amid the wars in Iraq and Afghanistan. Doctors, scientists and medical-based corporations have worked together to develop quick therapeutic and pain-relieving processes for our wounded troops.

Caught in the line of fire, these tried-and-true battlefield techniques have enabled military commanders to develop a system where severely wounded troops are extracted from battlefields as soon as possible. From there, our soldiers often are in operating rooms within a half hour after suffering horrendous injuries.

Working together, expert medical crews strive as soon as possible

71

to restore each wounded soldier's vital signs as soon as possible to optimal levels. Meantime, the soldiers in the battle zones and medical crews make the elimination of pain a top priority.

According to some news reports, at least 35,000 of the 1.65 million U.S. military service personnel deployed to Iraq and Afghanistan have been physically wounded. The advent and continued development of pain management teams should go a long way in addressing their physical and emotional pains. Despite the admirable advancements our military has made in the fight against physical pain, many of our soldiers, sailors and Air Force personnel have developed extreme addictions to the medications designed to fight such discomfort.

In January 2011, *USA Today* reported that one of our nations's most respected and highest-decorated three-star generals, Lt. Gen. David Fridovich, publicly admitted his own extreme addiction to pain killers. Standing before more than 700 of his personnel, Fridovich courageously acknowledged to his personal mistakes in this regard and urged the troops to use caution when administering pain killers to our military personnel. The general had been quietly hooked on pain killers during the previous five years.

Hospitalizations and diagnosis for substance abuse has doubled among members of the armed forces during the past decade. According to another *USA Today* article published the same day, from 25 percent to 35 percent of the 10,000 military personnel assigned to "wounded care companies or battalions are addicted to or dependant on drugs."

Such news comes as a sad, tragic development, especially to the many medical professionals—inside and outside of our military—who strive daily to legitimately and effectively eliminate the physical pains of others.

As a Vietnam Veteran and a retired U.S. Army National Guard Colonel, I applaud, admire and appreciate the courageous and admirable service of our troops in the Middle East and South Asia. Yet, just like Gen. Fridovich, I believe that our military can and should do more to confront and address the nagging problems of pain killer addictions among our troops.

First, the military should implement a better "command and control system" that involves the distribution and prescribing of pain killers. And second, the military needs to implement the use of well-controlled and carefully monitored natural human growth hormones, in order to speed up the natural healing process and thereby more quickly eliminate pain.

Chapter 5
'Wonder' Drugs
Emerge To Fight Pain

The generic, prevalent and often-effective substance we commonly call aspirin has been known to scientists since antiquity. Yet, amazingly, the vital, much-appreciated substance was not widely distributed and used until 1899 on the heels of the Spanish-American War the previous two years.

At seemingly the speed of light this so-called "wonder drug" engulfed the medical industry, while satisfying the urgent needs of individual consumers seeking relief from persistent and nagging aches and pains. By 1910, as the Industrial Revolution clicked into full gear, aspirin emerged as a common, accepted and expected feature of the American culture.

"Wine and cheese are like ageless companions, like aspirin and aches, or June and moon, or good people and noble virtues," said Mary Francis Kennedy Fisher, a widely acclaimed and respected 20th Century author.

Although scientists had known the many benefits of aspirin, comprised of willow bark extract, for more than 1,000 years, it wasn't until the mid-1800s that physicians began to fully appreciate and disseminate news of this substance's many wonderful qualities—particularly the ability to alleviate or eliminate pain, lessen fevers and relieve swelling.

Some historians believe that from 1803 to 1806 the explorers Meriwether Lewis and William Clark used willow bark extract to treat fevers during their famous exploration of western North America. From the mid- to late-1800s scientists experimented with and prescribed specific chemicals known as the active ingredients of willow bark. This research culminated in 1897, when the drug and dye firm Bayer worked with many of these researchers in devising methods of harnessing the active ingredients of the willow bark extracts.

In 1899 Bayer dubbed the resulting substance "aspirin." At the time the word was a brand name of the Bayer company, but the firm lost exclusive rights to produce and distribute the drug in numerous countries. In 1918 the popularity of aspirin skyrocketed when this amazing substance proved effective in relieving or at least addressing some symptoms during the worldwide flu pandemic that killed millions of people.

Aspirin Now a Basic Tool in Battling Pain

Even today, scientists and amazed physicians are discovering and appreciating the many stupendous benefits that aspirin can offer. Key among these is the ability to thin the blood, reducing the likelihood of death if taken at the onset of heart attacks. Some physicians swear to the irrefutable benefits of using typical aspirin as an anti-clotting agent, often effective as a preventative measure in battling cardiac problems and strokes.

All along, many of the world's largest, most greedy pharmaceutical companies undoubtedly dislike aspirin because it's relatively cheap for consumers and can easily be purchased at most pharmacies, grocery stores and convenience stores without prescriptions from physicians.

Thus, consumers seeking relief from basic pains or aches often can sidestep expensive visits to doctor's offices. As a result, Big Pharma misses out on at least some potential opportunities to gouge the public, the way these huge pharmaceutical companies do when charging $5 or much more for individual pain-killing pills other than aspirin.

Despite its many positive potential benefits, aspirin poses at least some possible drawbacks. The primary disadvantage occurs when aspirin causes or sets the stage for stomach upsets or ulcers, especially when taken if the person fails to eat immediately before or while ingesting these pills.

Aspirin also gets little or no attention from some people suffering from intense, super-uncomfortable pains because this generic product is much less powerful than many highly addictive substances. Still, aspirin remains a shining star within the realm of analgesics for the very reason that it's non-addictive on a physiological level. Of course, some people might take too much aspirin in an effort to satisfy their apparent psychological needs, but overall such problems seem rare and much less harmful than full-fledged pain-killing narcotics.

Aspirin's Role Remains Controversial

Even more than 100 years after the widespread emergence of aspirin historians remain at conflict as to which scientists played the most significant roles in contributing the Bayer company's efforts. Still, there is no denying that aspirin has played—and will continue to play—a significant and essential role in medicine.

This holds true even though numerous other over-the-counter or non-prescription pain-killers emerged for general purchases by consumers in the mid-1900s. These include acetaminophen introduced in 1956 and Ibuprofen launched just six years later, both listed as generally safe, low-power drugs with little harmful side effects when taken at suggested doses.

These developments gave the generic aspirin a run for its money, so to speak, during a period when some observers contend the overall popularity of the willow bark extract finally began to wane. Ever since then, scientists and particularly the research and development divisions of huge pharmaceutical companies have worked non-stop in efforts to discover or create new, effective low-range pain killers on the level of aspirin.

The emergence of acetaminophen and Ibuprofen came during a vastly different era of professionally acceptable marketing and promotions within the medical industry. During the years immediately after the official launch of aspirin, a vast array of medical professionals from doctors to hospital operators received packets of aspirin from Bayer—encouraging them to publish research papers on this drug.

When doctors began documenting and reporting positive results, Bayer continued efforts to patent and trademarks for aspirin. These efforts proved fruitless, however, because numerous companies had already begun producing and distributing aspirin by the time World War I erupted in 1914.

Even today, the specific ways that the various chemicals within aspirin actually generate positive symptoms remains in dispute. At first, some researchers and original developers of aspirin claimed that the willow tree bark derivative somehow blocked the transmission of pain signals from the nervous system to the brain. However, according to one published report, at least one researcher who used animals in tests concluded that aspirin's chemical compounds worked at the actual source of pain, such as a wound. While scientists continue to argue the specific reasons for aspirin's fantastic qualities, this low-cost drug will likely remain an essential tool in the pain-fighting analgesic category for many years.

Intravenous Therapy (IVs) Drastically Improved Delivery

Perhaps one of the greatest, most essential medical innovations as the Industrial Revolution reached full steam was intravenous therapy—commonly known as "IVs." At a steadily increasing pace starting in the late 1800s, these devices were used for a variety of methods of delivering vital fluids, drugs and eventually plasma to wounded or ill patients.

The IV devices entail the use of hypodermic needles or thin

catheters inserted into the patient's veins for the disbursement of vital, life-saving fluids, pharmaceuticals or even blood transfusions. For cases involving pain, intravenous devices give medical professionals and doctors the ability to quickly administer essential drugs or substances, particularly in life-threatening situations.

The use of IVs for specific uses from drug infusions to transfusions came in various phases through the 20th Century. From the start, the devices played essential roles in alleviating the pains and symptoms of dehydration, quickly re-hydrating the body following the extreme and life-threatening loss of essential fluids.

Just like doctors had done with aspirin, the medical industry quickly accepted the IV as an essential treatment tool. Physicians systematically accepted new and essential uses for intravenous therapy. This all became possible thanks to drip chambers that prevented air from entering the body's blood circulation systems.

Just like all other primary pharmaceuticals and medical devices, the IV units posed potential setbacks or complications to patients. Possible negative risks ranged from painful infection and phlebitis or swelling caused by such conditions. Other potential dangers from intravenous therapy include: fluid overload, putting excessive amounts of fluids into the body faster than it can absorb; hypothermia, when the body absorbs excessive levels of cold fluids; imbalances in the body's chemical levels or electrolytes; and potentially fatal embolisms, caused by delivery of blood clots, air bubbles or other solids.

While all these possible hazards are indeed serious, the countless benefits of intravenous therapy far outweigh the risks. In fact, during the first decade of my career in the 1970s as a full-time oncologist, I personally administered many chemotherapy treatments via IV to my cancer patients. Much of these laborious and complex chores needed my full attention, since my personal staff and hospital personnel levels lacked adequate numbers of certified, trained nurses or other medical professionals to handle all of those chores.

Medications developed independent of the military such as aspirin and the growing use of IVs were deployed to treat pain and wounds in World War I, World War II, the Korean War, the Vietnam War, the battle of Grenada, and the first Gulf War in the early 1990s.

Many pain-killing pharmaceuticals that consumers use today were initially administered at or during these conflicts. Especially in Vietnam in the 1960s and early 1970s, the military developed and honed the use of quickly delivering wounded soldiers via helicopter from battle zones to medical facilities or hospitals. Similar patient-delivery systems soon carried over into civilian life throughout the USA, enabling physicians to quickly treat pain, wounds or extreme illnesses such as heart attacks or strokes.

Addictive Morphine Entered Battlefields and General Medicine

Thanks largely to the increasingly common use of hypodermic needles and IVs, the extremely potent opiate morphine began making its way into battlefields to save wounded U.S. soldiers from the ravages of pain—particularly during the Vietnam War. The hypodermic needle, highly effective for the injection of drugs into the body, was actually invented in the 1850s.

Although initially used primarily by medical professionals, hypodermic needles were so specialized and easy to use that some drug addicts eventually became adept at administering their own hits. Like morphine, during the 1900s the hypodermic needle emerged as a double-edged sword, essential in the legitimate and necessary administering of medical treatments, and for the extremely harmful use by addicts as well. Composed of pointed, hallowed-out stainless steel tubes, hypodermic syringes became just as important to heroin addicts as to diabetics who needed to inject their own insulin.

Morphine gave many horribly injured U.S. soldiers just such a reason for hope, in many cases quickly blocking or masking painful sensations. Some physicians have even gone so far as to claim that morphine is the benchmark or even a gold standard among analgesics, thanks to its ability to relieve patients from intense suffering and extreme pain. But like other opiates made from opium, such as the dreadful drug heroin, morphine targets the body's central nervous system.

Doctors will be among the first people to tell you that morphine is so intense and effective at blocking painful sensations that—although some individuals can tolerate the substance—other persons can quickly become psychologically addicted. The actual physiological or biology-based addictions can take much longer to kick into full gear.

After their tours of duty or upon being discharged following medical treatment, some Vietnam War veterans returned to U.S.

society with debilitating addictions to morphine. For many, these
addictions progressed to heroin and other harmful narcotics.
More than ever before, and at an increasingly intense pace, the
many benefits and severe drawbacks of pain and of the increasing
number of medications to hinder that sensation spilled over into
the mainstream of popular American culture.

Morphine's Popularity Gradually Grew
for More Than 2,000 Years

Long before the Vietnam War, as far back as the early Byzantine
era 300 years after Christ, alchemists—specialists in transforming
metals—began tinkering to create early forms of morphine. More
than 1,200 years later in the early 1500s the Austrian alchemist,
botanist and physician Paracelsus wrote of a new highly potent
pain killer, an early precursor of morphine, but recommended its
use only on rare occasions.

The modern-day equivalent of morphine was discovered in 1804
by a German pharmacist, Friedrich Wilhelm Adam Sertürner.
Historians credit this creative genius with being the first person to
use opium in isolating the essential substances for morphine. By
some accounts, Sertürner named this new creation after the Greek
god Morpheus, hailed in mythology as "the god of dreams."

Thirteen years after Sertürner discovery, in 1817 a pharmaceutical
company began distributing morphine as an analgesic that also
could be used for treating alcoholism and even opium addiction.
Sales increased in both volume and geographic area through the
next several decades. However, by the time the Civil War erupted

in the early 1860s, scientists had begun to acknowledge that morphine was highly addictive.

"All sin tends to be addictive, and the terminal point of addiction is what is called damnation," said Wystan Hugh Auden, an early 20th Century English-born American dramatist, poet and editor. Indeed, according to some published accounts, many of 400,000 Civil War soldiers became addicted to morphine.

Bayer, the same company instrumental in initially launching and distributing aspirin, launched the widespread production and distribution of heroin in 1898, just 24 years after synthesizing that substance from morphine. Heroin got plenty of attention, hailed as about 2 ½ times more powerful than morphine and possessing an impressive capability of moving more easily from the blood to the brain.

Powerful Painkillers Became Illegal

The extreme addictiveness coupled with the mega-powerful potency of morphine motivated U.S. lawmakers to make possession of this substance illegal nationwide. With passage in 1914 of the Harrison Narcotics Tax Act, Congress outlawed this opiate-based substance unless accompanied by a prescription from a licensed physician. The law marked a significant social change—the banning of a powerful substance that much of the public yearned for, wanted and needed largely to fight pain. The very substances that people craved to fight extremely uncomfortable sensations became illegal unless used under medical supervision, and for a very good reason.

At the same time that technology advanced society's ability to discover, produce and distribute mass quantities of pain killers, people in many segments of the entire U.S. society experienced and suffered from the many negative side effects of narcotics. Besides opium-based products, the Harrison Narcotics Act imposed stiff restrictions on the production, distribution and possession of substances derived from cocoa leaves—the key ingredient in the highly addictive narcotic cocaine and once a primary ingredient in the earliest version of the popular soda, Coca-Cola.

Morphine, opium and heroin reigned as the most powerful and most frequently prescribed top-level, analgesic-class narcotic pain killers through most of the early 1900s. Just like aspirin had, morphine remained on the market for many years before physicians began to understand how its primary ingredients interact with the body.

Amazingly, according to a 2005 article "Human white blood cells synthesize morphine," scientists discovered that a specific receptor within the human body reacts only to this narcotic.

When used as an analgesic, doctors use morphine to relieve pain in certain types of medical conditions. The primary or most prevalent conditions are for:

- **Myocardial infractions:** Most commonly known as "heart attacks," these occur when the blood supply to the heart gets interrupted, resulting in an extremely painful condition.

- **Sickle-cell crisis:** These conditions caused by a blood disorder sometimes result in extreme pain, when certain cells lose flexibility and thereby generate complications.

- **Extreme conditions:** These pains occur as a result of everything from trauma caused by car wrecks and war wounds to conditions resulting from surgery.

- **Chronic pain:** This long-term or persistent condition results from such relentless debilitating conditions as cancer, kidney stones or severe muscular-skeletal injuries or diseases.

Morphine is also sometimes used for a variety of other conditions, or in conunction with other drugs, for everything from severe coughs to an adjunct to general anesthesia, and even for a chronic diarrhea associated with AIDS.

This drug is most often administered via IV, but other methods include orally, via injection, or inhaling—a method commonly used by abusers. Even when used in antibacterial-free medical environments, morphine can result in serious medical complications such as addiction, constipation, and the unintentional transmission of harmful viruses in instances where blood or other substances are not adequately checked beforehand.

Although a potentially dangerous and highly addictive narcotic, morphine can serve a legitimate and often-necessary role in the world's non-stop battle against physical pain. In my personal and professional view, this often misunderstood substance should remain available as a vital potential tool in the medical industry's battle to give patients relief and thereby opening a pathway for potential recovery.

The so-called big brother or master of morphine is the naturally growing and highly dangerous substance opium. Highly addictive, this plant has been used since the Stone Age and then by such societies as the early Romans.

Used as the primary ingredient for the deadly and highly addictive heroin, opium is so powerful that just 12 percent of it contains the primary effective ingredients of morphine. More than 500 years ago the Chinese recognized opium's tremendous power, as various segments of that society began adopting the drug for recreational use.

"Among the remedies which it has pleased Almighty God to give man to relieve his sufferings, none is so universal and so efficacious as opium," said Thomas Sydenham, a 17th Century English physician. Such observations may have hit the proverbial bull's-eye dead center from the medical aspect, yet there can be no denying that opium has generated various sufferings for humanity, from severe addictions, to wrecked personal finances and broken families. Once again, with opium we see we must come to grips with the fact that the best, most effective pain killers also can create great harm.

"Nobody will laugh long who deals much with opium; its pleasures even are of a grave and solemn complexion," said Thomas de Quincey, a 19th Century English author and intellectual who wrote "Confessions of an English Opium-Eater" in 1821.

The opium trade became such an important economic force for the British Empire that from 1839 to 1858 during the "Opium Wars" the Europeans strived to continue distribution of the substance in China despite its emperor's ban on such commerce. Opium poppies are grown and harvested predominantly in Southern Asia including vastly divergent nations like India and Afghanistan. Archaeologists also have found evidence of opium use long ago in Spain, Switzerland and Germany.

Researchers say that the use, distribution and trade of opium became so prevalent more than 1,000 years ago that the drug spread into the early Greek, Mediterranean and European cultures. Within the Persian area of the Middle East some physicians began using opium to treat melancholy and as an anesthetic.

"Opium teaches only one thing, which is that aside from physical suffering, there is nothing real," said Andre Malreaux, an award-winning 20th Century author, statesman and French adventurer.

Opium Blasted into the Mainstream Culture

Opium had become such a mainstay within the European and eventually the American medical culture that—by some accounts—it was among substances used to treat U.S. President William Henry Harrison after he contracted a fatal bout of pneumonia in March 1841. The ninth U.S. president, he became the first of our nation's chief executives to die in office, 32 days after his inauguration.Some historians have claimed that opium treatments worsened Harrison's physical condition along with fruitless efforts to use leeches and castor oil.

According to a 2008 issue of the *American Journal of Pharmaceutical Education*, during the Civil War the Union Army issued what—at least to me—seemed like a mind-boggling, staggering 500,000 opium pills, and 2.8 million ounces of opium tincture.

By today's medical standards, at least from my professional view, such widespread distribution of the drug was highly dangerous from a societal standpoint. Yet rather than sharply criticizing those efforts, we should remain cognizant that for the most part many physicians were merely administering what they considered the best-available pain remedies for their era.

"The expense of a war could be paid in time; but the expense of opium, when once the habit is formed, will only increase with time," said Townsend Harris, a New York merchant and a minor politician in the 1800s.

By some estimates up to three-fourths of the 150,000-200,000 opiate addicts in the United States in the late 19th Century were women—most of whom received opium as a prescription for female-related medical situations such as menstrual pain.

During the final decades of the 19th Century American communities began recognizing the ravages of opium, placing legal restrictions on the drug. By 1919, tough regulations spread throughout California and eventually nationwide.

Opium-based Pain Killers Reigned Supreme

Throughout the early 20th Century painkillers derived from opium or synthetic versions of that substance remained the most effective drugs for painkilling. This ignited and spread the overwhelming and extremely dangerous potential for life-changing addictions.

The advent of synthetic opiates failed to stem this tide, such as the 1957 introduction of methadone and fentany. Despite these advancements, the U.S. military's combat medics still preferred to carry morphine. Perhaps largely for this reason, morphine is still legally produced in various nations primarily in Asia and South America. Despite the U.S. involvement in a war against the Taliban in Afghanistan, that nation remains the world's top illegal producer of poppies for the eventual production of heroin smuggled into the United States and Europe.

Meantime, the demand for opium for legitimate medicinal reasons including the production of morphine became so intense that in 2006 a drug company received permission from Britain to legally harvest poppies in that region. In a sense the so-called battle between good and evil get intermixed and confused, since drug abusers and legitimate users of opiate-based pharmaceuticals continue to show strong worldwide demand.

Scientists Developed a Vast Array of Analgesics

Backed by research and scientific developments through thousands of years and many wars, 20th Century physicians helped create and embraced a vast array of pain-killing pharmaceuticals called "analgesics." For the most part these are comprised of opium-based products such as morphine, and also salicylate or salicylic acid-based products derived from willow tree bark.

In a majority of cases, physicians choose specific analgesics depending on the diagnosed severity of pain stemming from specific types of wounds or illnesses. Yet, analgesics are not effective for all types of pain, such as instances of neuropathic pain that occur as a result of certain types of lesions, specific disorders within the peripheral nervous system such as in the spinal cord or brain, or in specific types of cancers. Other potential factors include complications following chemotherapy, diabetic neuropathies, and post-herpetic neuropathy.

Medications within the general spectrum of analgesics are not designed to cover all types of physical pain. In addition, it is also important for patients to remember that the analgesic category should not be confused with anesthetics—pharmaceuticals administered only by medical professionals to eliminate sensations during major surgeries or for much less serious medical procedures such as dentistry, the removal of toenails by podiatrists or minor surgical procedures such as colonoscopies.

Patients who want to know the basics of the analgesic category of choices often find it useful to understand the primary classes or subsets within this realm. They are:

- **Paracetamol**: Also known as NSAIDs, these are non-steroidal and anti-inflammatory drugs like aspirin. As an overall category, paracetamol generates fewer side-effects than much more powerful analgesics, while also usually lacking the propensity for dangerous addictions. Despite extensive advances in overall science, researchers still fail to understand how this substance works in all instances. Numerous studies indicate these substances work centrally within the brain rather than on nerve endings. Despite its ranking as relatively safe compared to much more powerful analgesics, overuse of paracetamol can damage the upper gastrointestinal tract, the liver, or generate a variety of physical problems such as hearing loss, kidney damage and allergic reactions. In addition, especially among children, suffering from Reye's Syndrome fever, a severe allergy to aspirin that can cause potentially fatal brain and liver disease.

- **COX-2 Inhibitors:** Developed largely by pharmaceutical companies, these are generally derived from the same substances used to create aspirin, created largely in an effort to block specific types of enzymes in order to develop less gastrointestinal hemorrhaging. This compares to aspirin, which sometimes causes stomach ulcerations or digestive tract problems, especially when ingested regularly on an empty stomach. Despite the advantages of COX-2 inhibitors, this substance also poses an array of potential physical setbacks, according to various published reports. These include the possibility of cardiac problems or CNS disorders. COX-2 inhibitors have also been used in the treatment of colorectal cancers as adjuvant therapies.

- **Opiates:** Also including morphine and various other drugs, this is among the most powerful but potentially addictive range within analgesics. Despite the extremely powerful pain-killing attributes within the opiate and

morphinomimetics range, this class can result in many
potentially unpleasant side effects. Besides the risk
of itching and constipation, these drugs also pose the
potential problems of vomiting and nausea. Thus, many
physicians also prescribe additional medications such
as laxatives when treating patients with this type of
analgesic. Some of the most common drugs within the
opiate and morphine-based category are:

- **Codeine:** Extracted from opium poppies, this is
  generally considered within the weak or mid-range
  level of the opiate class. The specific ingredients
  of codeine are made from only a small portion
  of the numerous active ingredients from the
  poppies. According to at least some published
  accounts, codeine has just 8 percent to 12 percent
  of the overall pain-fighting strength of morphine.
  Usually taken orally as a pill, codeine is often
  considered less addictive than morphine and is
  most often prescribed for mild or moderate pain.
  Codeine is sometimes sold under brand names
  such as Vicodin when intermixed with lower-dose
  acetaminophen. The potential adverse effects of
  codeine can include everything from euphoria,
  depression and constipation to nausea, drowsiness,
  itching, rashes, and other complications.

- **Oxycodone**: Also primarily comprised from a
  specific active ingredient produced by opium
  poppies, this is categorized as a "semi-synthetic"
  because the drug is produced when compounding

isolated substances from within natural sources. Sometimes sold under the time-released brand name OxyContin produced by Purdue Pharma—the rights remaining under dispute—this also is available in generic form. Historians of drug research say scientists in Germany discovered or isolated oxycodone in 1916, and scientists subsequently achieved at least some of their objective of generating this as a less-addictive alternative to heroin. Under the brand name OxyContin, use increased sharply from the mid-1990s through the first decade of the 21st Century, and according to news reports the manufacturer changed the formula in 2010 in attempts to decrease misuse of this drug. In recent years, the news media has reported various marketing and branding issues involving OxyContin. Meantime, at least seven other brand names with varying related compounds have been marketed and distributed. Besides euphoria and memory loss, the various potential side effects of oxycodone can include everything from nausea and constipation to dizziness and headaches, plus anxiety and more intense side effects of codeine.

● **Hydrocodone**: Also a semi-synthetic and derived from opium, as a specific ingredient found within the poppies, this pain killer is often taken in the form of a tablet or as a syrup to depress coughs. Some scientists debate the effectiveness of hydrocodone, particularly when taken without other analgesics. Nonetheless, at least judging by

some published accounts, hydrocodone might be
at least two times more effective than standard
codeine. First approved by the FDA in 1943 for
U.S. sales, initially under the brand name Hycocan,
hydrocodone eventually got manufactured,
distributed and sold under at least 20 brand names.
Although deemed stronger than codeine but with
only one tenth of morphine's strength, this drug
poses the potential of harmful addiction. As a
result, physicians sometimes prescribe this only
under strict supervision with drugs designed to
counteract some potentially harmful effects, or with
other analgesics. Used for mild to moderate pain,
hydrocodone can generate severe negative reactions
when mixed with certain other drugs like alcohol,
barbiturates or cocaine. Its side effects include all of
those sometimes generated by codeine.

- **Dihydromorphine**: Physicians describe this as
very similar to morphine, sometimes even stronger
than that drug—acting faster and lasting longer.
Also an opiate, this semi-synthetic was discovered
in 1900, at least a generation before some of its
less powerful counterparts. Partly as a result of
this drug's extreme strength, the U.S. government
considers dihydromorphine as an extremely
dangerous "Schedule 1" narcotic. Its specific
strength when compared to morphine, whether
less or more effective, remains in dispute among
researchers. It is marketed under the name Dilaudid.

- **Pethidine**: Commonly called "Demerol," but also referred to by a wide variety of other names, this opiate analgesic is sometimes termed as a "meperidine." Heralded as fast-acting and first introduced in 1932, this was considered as the opiate that many physicians preferred when prescribing opium-based medications during much of the 20th Century. But perhaps because some physicians consider pethidine as no more effective than morphine, this drug decreased in popularity while being severely restricted in some countries such as Australia. Considered highly addictive, its possible severe potential side effects include tremors, seizures, and "dysphoria," a term for uncontrollably unpleasant moods. This analgesic is seldom used in oncology.

- **Flupirtine**: While not an opiate, unrelated to willow tree barks, and not steroid-based, this drug first introduced by Asta Medica in Europe in 1984 for pain treatment has never been introduced in the United States. In 2008, the Adeona pharmacy acquired an option to license the pending and issued patents for Flupirtine, while scientists research its possible effectiveness as a treatment for Alzheimer's Disease, multiple sclerosis, and fibromyalgia, a medical disorder that results in muscular and connective tissue pain.

- **Other specific agents**: In addition to the aspirin-like and opiate-based drugs in the analgesic category, a variety of other substances are sometimes either used or considered. These might include specific types of anti-depressants or tricyclic antidepressants. In most instances, as the description implies, this is used to relieve the symptoms of depression. Meantime, certain anti-depressants are sometimes also prescribed for the treatment of chronic pain. Nefopam™, first developed as an opiate alternative in the early 1970s, is widely used but mostly in Europe. Much stronger at fighting pain than aspirin, Nefopam sometimes causes sweating, dizziness and nausea, while deemed half as potent as oxycodone and morphine.

Chapter 6

Anesthesia Drugs and Steroids Become Pain Fighters

Patients who undergo anything from a basic outpatient procedure such as dental work to extensive surgery usually require an anesthetic, sometimes spelled "anaesthetic." For the most part these drugs create what doctors call the "reversible loss of sensation."

Except for extreme or rare instances, anesthetic pharmaceuticals are not used to deaden or block pain during non-surgical periods. For less extensive procedures, licensed professionals such as dentists working on teeth or podiatrists extracting toenails administer lower-dose anesthetics during outpatient procedures performed in their clinics.

For many of the most complex procedures, surgeons often work with the assistance of specialized anesthesiologists. Such licensed and highly educated professionals administer specific types of powerful anesthetics. When administered correctly, powerful anesthetics used in surgeries put the patient in a sleep-like state for

96

a limited period. Extremely serious complications and even death can occur if such drugs are administered incorrectly, or when such patients fail to receive continuous monitoring by a certified anesthesiologist.

Authorities say the abuse of high-powered anesthetics is extremely rare, largely due to the extreme danger involved. Perhaps the most famous case of such apparent abuse involved the late entertainment superstar Michael Jackson, at least according to criminal prosecutors. Jackson died at age 50 in June 2009 in what the Los Angeles Coroner's Office listed as a homicide involving a powerful anesthetic. Jackson's personal physician, Conrad Murray, pleaded not guilty to criminal manslaughter charges. News stories quoted Jackson's acquaintances as saying the restless star abused analgesics in order to get much-needed sleep.

The Jackson case should serve as an urgent example to all sufferers of intense pain that they should never consider or try any form of anesthetic in an attempt to administer at-home relief for sleep problems. Even physicians say the in-home use of such powerful anesthetics is ill-advised, extremely dangerous and unnecessary, even when administered by a doctor. For patients suffering from sleep problems, physicians have a wide range of other much more sensible treatments or lifestyle changes.

Anesthetics Fall within Specified Classifications

Pharmacists and medical professionals list anesthetics within two primary classifications. The first, "general anesthetics," puts patients in a temporary unconsciousness during significant medical procedures such as surgery. The "local anesthetics" category generates a temporary loss of sensation in a specific part of the body while patients remain awake.

In addition to general and local anesthetics, the anesthesia branch of medicine features two additional classifications that are not often in the public mindset. The first of these is "regional anesthetics" where an entire section of the body such as a limb is treated to induce a loss of sensation. Doctors sometimes use a catheter to continuously inject anesthetic drugs into a specific area of the body, such as epidural procedures performed upon the onset of childbirth's final stage, or for a caesarian section.

Medical experts consider the application of regional anesthetics as potentially more dangerous than local anesthetics that are done in extremely limited bodily areas such as the fingers, toes or teeth. Possible complications from regional procedures include seizures, cardiac arrest or spinal shock where many physical sensations are blocked for extended periods.

Due to these possible dangers, in case of a medical emergency, physicians performing regional procedures such as localized operations on limbs are sometimes prepared to immediately revert to general anesthesia impacting the entire body.

As a result of these dangers, many regional anesthetic procedures like extensive facelift operations are done in extremely safe conditions. Although such surgeries are often performed within a doctor's office, such facilities frequently provide highly trained personnel capable of administering general anesthetics.

For minor procedures that need local anesthetics, medical

professionals have a choice from at least ten substances that block the ability of nerves to transmit the sensation of pain. Many doctors prefer to avoid three of these options because they are considered unstable while also often resulting in allergic reactions—cocaine, procaine and amethocaine. This leaves the remaining options, each ending in the phrase "caine," indicating that the effective substances render cellular communications or interactions via the nervous system, rendering those sections of the body ineffective for limited periods.

In both general anesthetics and local anesthetics the term "anesthesia" is used to describe what occurs when the doctor intentionally induces either of three reversible states or conditions:

- **Amnesia**: A temporary loss of memory.

- **Analgesia**: The temporary elimination of responsiveness from sensations including pain, while also decreasing skeletal muscle reflexes and responses to stress.

- **Multi-effects**: A variety of some, or all, of the above-listed temporary outcomes.

Before any scheduled medical procedures requiring local or general anesthetics, patients should feel free to ask questions about how the surgery is performed.

Dissociative Anesthetics Impact the Mental Process

Besides local, general and regional anesthetics, doctors also sometimes use "dissociative anesthetics" in a specified effort to block or curtail the transmission of pain signals from the conscious mind to various areas of the brain.

Many of these narcotics, some of them addictive, produce hallucinogenic effects. The related possible side effects range from sensory deprivation to trances or "dream-like states," and even a sense of dissociation—when the mind feels distanced from the physical realm. The level, duration and occurrence of these specific conditions are often unpredictable and challenging for almost any physician to foresee.

These behaviors or reactions sometimes strike patients and even seasoned medical professionals who care for them as rather unsettling. Some patients, even those striving to fight off pain, end up behaving in unanticipated ways far different from their usual lifestyle patterns.

Besides intentionally via the use of narcotics or anesthetics, the occurrence of dissociative mental reactions sometimes erupts as a result of trauma or mental abuse. Such causes increase the complexity of challenging symptoms among patients recovering from such trauma as gunshot wounds or sexual attacks.

Most doctors avoid prescribing psychoactive drugs in any attempt to alleviate or block physical pain. The many substances that generate dissociative properties can range from LSD and alcohol to PCP and atropine—all within the category of psychoactive drugs. Despite the many potential drawbacks, such substances sometimes result in blocking or warding off extreme physical or emotional pain.

Numerous pharmaceutical companies use derivatives from plants around the world to generate anesthetic drugs accepted and used by mainstream physicians. Although known today primarily as a highly addictive and extremely dangerous narcotic, in the mid-1800s cocaine was sometimes used as an anesthetic.

After inhaled or inhalational anesthetics such as diethyl ether were first introduced in 1846—initially for dentistry—and chloroform, many of the anesthetic drugs used most frequently today for a wide variety of medical procedures were gradually approved by the medical industry during the following 150 years.

The emergence of these new life-saving technologies gradually resulted in the increasingly accepted and even the required medical specialty of anesthesiologists. These highly trained medical professionals devote their careers to providing and implementing anesthetics in the safest conditions possible. According to a 2010 report by the American Society of Anesthesiologists, of the more than 40 million annual medical procedures requiring anesthetics, such professionals provided or administered anesthetic in 90 percent of the cases.

In the United States, in order to become fully certified, anesthesiologists must undergo at least four years of residency or post-graduate medical training in their specialty—starting after they graduate from medical school. Thus, like general physicians and highly specialized practices such as oncology, these professionals must excel through a minimum combined 12 years of college and post-graduate education after high school.

In addition, in the United States some hospitals or medical

facilities also employ "certified registered nurse anesthetists" or CRNAs. Many of these nurses work for anesthesiologists, hospitals, surgeons, podiatrists, dentists, obstetricians and other medical professionals who regularly render anesthetics.

Increasingly during the 20th Century and particularly during the past several decades, anesthetics has become so specialized and essential to the success of overall medical care that many facilities also employ "anesthesia technicians." In much the way that scrub technicians assist surgeons, an anesthesia technician performs essential duties for anesthesiologists.

As seen in popular TV shows and in the movies, high-level anesthetic equipment features extensive, complex and often essential machines ranging from vaporizers to pressure gauges and ventilators. A malfunction of any or all of these devices could result in a medical emergency, such as the break of a vital machine part or the unintentional transmission of harmful bacteria to the patient—risking serious or even fatal infections.

Adding to the complexity, throughout extensive medical procedures and surgeries anesthesiologists are responsible for continually monitoring a patient's vital signs. All essential bodily functions are tracked, from the heart rate to blood pressure, EKG and EEG monitoring, oxygen levels, and the intake or output of gasses.

As if these many urgent tasks weren't already enough in the overall process of blocking pain, the vast team of doctors and nurses depends on anesthesiologists to monitor pressures within blood vessels. When any of these vital signs malfunctions, these doctors work with the entire medical crew to re-stabilize the patient. Seasoned and well-trained professionals take these responsibilities in stride, responding to specific types of emergencies in pre-defined, step-by-step manners—following an exact protocol.

Some Patients Remain Alert and Aware
of Pain During Surgery

Shockingly, at least judging by numerous stories in recent years in the mainstream news media, some patients who underwent surgery claimed they remained fully alert and feeling intense pain during their operations. Some observers have termed this condition as "anesthesia awareness" or "unintended intra-operative awareness."

In at least some cases, patients claim that medical professionals failed to give them enough anesthetic to render them fully unconscious during surgery. Could many of these patients be confused, wrongly believing that what they sensed while regaining consciousness in the recovery room had actually occurred during their surgeries?

Beginning early in this century, some published reports have estimated that from 0.01% to 0.02%, or about one or two out of every thousand people who undergo surgery, claim to have remained in a state of awareness during the procedure.

Once again, here, I feel a need to state my professional opinion. Reports of such instances need much more study before physicians can make any conclusive statements on the issue. Before any of my patients undergoes surgery, if they might happen to inquire, I would tell them that any instance of anesthesia awareness remains extremely unlikely. For more than a century, anesthesiologists have developed pre-specified systems of determining the amount of drugs needed to render a person fully unconscious—largely dependant on the person's body weight and overall physical structure.

Also on the positive side, only about one third to nearly one half of those who claim to remain aware during surgery reported that they felt any pain, at least judging by some published reports. Understandably, nearly all of those who claimed to have felt pain—a full 94 percent of them—claimed that they suffered from anxiety or panic, in some instances experiencing difficulty breathing.

Patients commonly remain awake during local anesthesia for minor in-office, outpatient surgeries. A much less common practice occurs when physicians intentionally keep the patient awake during some major operations.

During some brain operations, for instance, surgeons strive to keep patients fully cognizant during the procedures in order to signal to doctors what they feel—if anything—when a specific part of the body gets touched. These procedures also can serve as an essential way for the patient to communicate, or to specify whether various regions of the body are functioning as planned.

Steroids Also Play a Huge Role

Much mainstream media publicity about steroids focuses on the illegal, ill-advised or dangerous use of such substances by athletes. However, many people fail to realize steroids also can play a vital role in legitimate medicine, particularly in eradicating painful conditions.

Steroids get a much-deserved bad rap because many of these substances are known carcinogens. However, when used in prescribed medical conditions under a doctor's supervision, steroids can alleviate or lessen painful conditions such as certain lung problems, muscular diseases or arthritis conditions.

Steroids are either synthetically created by pharmaceutical companies, or they are derived from plants. Within the human body, steroids occur naturally. Part of the problem that steroids pose stems from the fact that when used as drugs they're administered in highly concentrated amounts, often far more than the body normally uses.

The human body naturally generates many types of hormones, such as sex hormones that regulate everything from the libido to reproductive tendencies.

Some hormones also possess anti-inflammatory characteristics, often ideal for eliminating painful symptoms. Nonetheless, steroids also can emerge as highly destructive within the bodies of athletes striving to artificially build or retain muscle mass.

Besides features affecting sexual functions and cholesterol levels, within the class of vertebrate steroids that impact creatures with backbones there are two integral subsets involving pain:

- **Anabolic steroids**: These impact the muscles, sex organs, and bones, hinging on androgen receptors by using natural or synthetic substances.

- **Corticosteroids**: These impact everything from stress

levels to immune system responses, levels of inflammation and behavior, including "fight or flight" responses.

Due to the extreme power and potential dangers of these substances, the possession and use of many specific types of anabolic steroids and corticosteroids in drug form is illegal unless under the prescription of a licensed physician. A patient seeking relief of pain should never under any circumstances attempt to obtain and use such substances outside of a doctor's care. Besides cancer, the potential life-threatening or debilitating long-term consequences of corticosteroids include cataracts, insulin resistant diabetes mellitus, permanent eye damage from glaucoma, depression, anxiety, muscle weakness, immune suppression, central obesity and "striate," commonly known as "stretch marks."

Within the corticosteroid class, synthetic glucocorticoids are often used in legitimate medicine to relieve debilitating conditions that cause joint pain and inflammation—most notably arthritis, dermatitis, asthma, cancers, and many other ailments.

Cortisone Enabled Physicians to Hit a Grand Slam Against Pain

Thanks largely to the isolation of cortisone made possible in part by the significant contributions of Edward Kendall, a researcher at the Mayo Clinic, Merck & Company began producing cortisone in the 1950s. As the end-product of an extensive, complex biological process that involves the adrenal glands, the body produces "cortisol," a natural response to stress that increasing blood sugar levels. Meantime, while suppressing the immune system, cortisol also assists in various metabolism functions that involve carbohydrates, fats and proteins.

Scientists list cortisone as an inactive metabolite of cortisol. When produced naturally within the body, cortisone serves as nature's way of reacting to stress. This is the same process that erupts during an extreme emergency, such as when the body prepares for a "flight or fight" mode, sometimes giving people extreme and unexpected strength in running away from their adversaries or even in order to battle their opponents.

Doctors sometimes employ this technique, generating short-term pain relief by injecting cortisone directly into an affected or swollen joint or tendon such as the knee, shoulder and elbow. Patients who had suffered extreme, excruciating pain in those areas often proclaim that cortisone is a "miracle" immediately after receiving such treatments.

"My knee had hurt so bad that I once couldn't walk or move," said Patricia, a patient who recently received cortisone for her persistent condition. "Right after the shot, everything was better right away and the pain subsided."

Like many other patients, Patricia also was advised to take pro-active lifestyle changes in order to treat her underlying condition. Thereafter, at least five days a week she exercised in the swimming pool of an exercise facility, and the pain never returned for several years. But her knee pain slowly began to re-emerge after a necessary operation to remove an ingrown toenail; the recovery period from that procedure prevented her from engaging in her favorite exercise routine for more than one month.

Understandably, Patricia resumed her exercise regimen as soon as possible, once again enabling her knee pain to subside. Her story serves as just one example that short-term pain killing remedies such as cortisone should not be considered as the only solution to eradicating pain. Ultimately, when working under the advice of their patients, many patients suffering from chronic pain need to engage in consistent physical therapy or vital and consistent exercise routines.

Meantime, cortisone should never be considered as the one-and-only drug for treating such pains. Like all other potentially powerful medications or substances, this steroid derivative poses numerous negative side effects due to its impact on the immune system. Potential myocardial arrests and excessive fluid in the abdomen are among dangers.

Anabolic Steroids Remain Highly Controversial

Another subset within this class, anabolic steroids, remains highly controversial due to the extreme dangers involved, coupled with use by professional athletes.

While mirroring the effects of male sex hormones such as testosterone, anabolic steroids generate masculine qualities like excessive hair, deepened voices and expansive muscles.

Since scientists first identified, isolated and began creating synthetic versions of anabolic steroids in the 1930s, the controversy has stirred and never seems to subside. Just some of the many potential dangerous side effects when used long-term include damage to the heart's left ventricle and severe or life-threatening liver damage.

As mentioned in several of my other best-selling books, including one endorsed by superstar media personality Suzanne Somers, some of the world's most popular sports heroes have abused anabolic steroids to get a competitive edge. Even before researchers isolated these substances, called "gonadal steroids," in the 1800s physicians began studying extracts from the testicles. In the late 1930s, bodybuilders and weightlifters were among the first athletes to begin abusing anabolic steroids.

Covertly, many athletes liked the way these steroids generated proteins to increase muscle mass, while also blocking the negative impacts of stress on muscles. When used under careful and authorized medical supervision, anabolic steroids can help improve or relieve the painful side effects of such ailments as osteoporosis and traumas caused by surgeries or extensive periods of remaining motionless.

Meantime, doctors and their patients need to remain aware of the potential adverse psychiatric effects, which can include mood disorders and substance abuse. Highly aggressive behaviors sometimes occur, often called "roid rage" that has been known to result in manic characteristics, physically abusive behavior, and even suicide.

Despite these many undeniable problems, physicians have used anabolic steroids for lots of specific pain-related treatments with varying degrees of success. Besides treating various forms of aneimas, other conditions include arthritis, kidney failure, leukemia, and breast cancer; these substances can also stimulate growth and appetite.

Even in the midst of such potential benefits, virtually every significant professional sports organization bans the use of anabolic steroids, including Major League Baseball, the National Football League and the National Basketball Association.

Chapter 7

Drastic Pain Relief Measures
Require Caution

A cvital medical specialty commonly called neurology often performs an important role in the detection, diagnosis and potential elimination of pain. Practicing neurologists focus on any disorder within the body's entire nervous structures—the autonomic, central and peripheral nervous systems.

Since the nervous system plays an essential role in communicating the signals of pain from various areas of the body to the brain, neurologists often are sought after as a first-line of analysis, diagnosis and detection as they devise and implement treatments. The role of neurologists in pain-related specialties within standard medicine handle everything from performing or managing research for pharmaceutical companies to conducting clinical trials of current or proposed painkillers. All these many tasks involve "neuroscience," the science and study of the body's nervous system.

Besides pain-related medical conditions such as gunshot wounds or even the ravages of advanced arthritis, these physicians often

identify and treat many types of neurological disorders. These
range from paralysis to muscle weaknesses, to seizures and other
adverse characteristics that often result in extreme pain. Many of
these problems stem from chemical or electrical abnormalities,
some inherited. According to various published reports, the World
Health Organization has estimated that at least 1 billion people,
or nearly one out of every seven people has at least one type of
neurological disorder.

People suffering from strange or seemingly unexplainable pains
often get their first definitive "answers" about their conditions
after finally seeing a neurologist. Many problems stem from
abnormalities within the brain, spinal cord or nervous systems.

Thankfully, once a neurologist has located and specified a specific
nerve-related cause to a painful disorder, he or she can then seek
to issue the best-possible treatments. Possible adverse conditions
or symptoms include migraine headaches, sleep disorders and
certain types of back pain. Some neurologists choose to specialize
in any of a vast range of disorders, such as dementia, epilepsy and
multiple sclerosis.

Physicians Disable the Spinal Cord in Extreme Cases

Certain severe, excruciatingly painful medical instances motivate
physicians to undertake the extraordinary procedure of disabling
sections of the spinal cord. Specifically, this process called a
"cordotomy" involves a surgical procedure where specific pain-
conducting tracts within the spinal cord are disabled.

In layman's terms, the cordotomy procedures are usually done as a last resort in cases where a patient is terminally ill with inoperable afflictions such as highly advanced prostate cancer, or for a variety of incurable diseases.

Such specific and complex surgeries, often performed as a humanitarian measure to relieve a patient of extreme pain during life's final stage, usually are performed with a needle rather than by opening the body with a scalpel. During a cordotomy, the patient usually does not feel pain in the area of the operation thanks to a local anesthetic.

Amid the procedure, the surgeon often uses a fluoroscopy device that enables the viewing of the body's internal structures. However, the procedure poses potential risks, primarily because in certain instances the patient gets exposed to consistent but low doses of radiation—a known carcinogen.

Before undergoing a cordotomy the physician considers the risks to the patient when matched to the urgent need to eliminate pain— plus the person's overall current condition. Also, for the most part, physicians usually recommend a cordotomy to a patient only after treatments in the highest level of the ladder of pain, primarily opium-derived drugs, have failed to get adequate results.

Other high-level, final-resort procedures to eliminate excruciating and chronic pain sometimes involve what doctor's call "nerve ablation"—literally the removal of that organ from the body. Most ablations involve procedures that do not attempt to relieve pain, such as facelifts or the removal of wrinkled skin, or even deadening certain areas of the atria via electrical frequencies in attempts to abolish abnormal heartbeats.

When targeting pain, the nerve ablation process can entail removing a specific wounded or damaged area of the body, or taking out a section of the brain that senses the discomfort. Some neurological disorders such as Parkinson's disease sometimes result in doctors recommending the removal of certain areas of the brain.

Much of the time the ablation of nerves or tumors is done via lasers with varying degrees of intensity. While minimally invasive to the body, such procedures are sometimes called "radio frequency ablation."

In addition to the removal of small-sized body parts or nerves in efforts to eliminate pain, doctors also sometimes must resort to the amputation of entire limbs. Amputations are usually done only in extreme cases, not usually for the specific purpose of relieving pain, but primarily due to the deadening, or to an extreme and irreversible disfiguring of the limb.

Abuse of Addictive Drugs Compound the Problem

Greedy hospitals and physicians in countries outside North America are compounding the pain relief problem, in conjunction with money-hungry U.S.-based drug companies.

An increasingly steady number of news reports in recent years have described how low-paid doctors in countries such as China over-prescribe pain drugs and antibiotic medications. According to a February 2011 article in *USA Today*,"this problem occurs because the compensation for usually low-paid doctors in China is based on how much revenue they generate.

As a result, in an effort to increase their own pay, many of these physicians sometimes issue pain medications or other drugs delivered via IV drips, although in many cases these treatments are unnecessary. Compounding the problems, pharmaceutical companies allegedly issue kickbacks to low-paid Chinese doctors who are willing to issue prescriptions for the corporation's drugs.

Adding more heartache to this corrupt system, some unsuspecting patients who receive pain killers and other drugs experience severe overdoses and critical medical complications. Across China and numerous other nations where entire societies are just beginning to benefit from advancements in medical technology, the responsibility goes to "barefoot doctors"—such as farmers who once learned the rudimentary basics of medicine.

On an international scale, the overall ongoing battle by the entire human population in fighting physical pain is complex, prone to corruption, and failing patients.

As a result, I strongly urge physicians everywhere, and especially the large drug companies, to work in the best interest of each patient. Doctors everywhere need to remind themselves to adhere to the Hippocratic Oath, which all physicians take when entering the profession, promising to practice medicine in an ethical manner.

Far from being a holier-than-thou statement on my part, such mindful and clear-cut objectives should remain at the forefront of physicians everywhere. This adherence to a supreme ethical standard also should hold fast throughout the upcoming advancements in pain-fighting technology.

Unethical Sales of Pain Pills Produce Controversy

The controversy of painkiller abuse got national attention in February 2011, when police and federal agents barged into the South Florida offices of doctors suspected of over-prescribing highly addictive pain killers like Oxycodone.

Authorities seized literally dozens of exotic cars in the raids, which resulted in the arrests of at least 22 people including physicians. The U.S. Drug Enforcement Agency, commonly called the "DEA," joined police in calling the operations "pill mills."

While authorities allege such illegal operations thrive nationwide, these enterprises have excelled at an astounding rate across Florida far more than any other state. Various news media reports said that purchases of oxycodone in Florida surpassed the purchases of the same drug in all states combined during the first half of 2010. Amazingly, however, Florida was among states that lack programs to monitor these pervasive drug pipelines; the Sunshine State's Republican governor at the time, Rick Scott, had been quoted as saying that such an effort would be too expensive and an invasion of privacy.

Investigators claim that operators of these cash-only clinics conducted only cursory medical examinations before the facilities' physicians issued prescriptions for narcotic pain killers. A DEA spokesman, Rusty Payne, told the news media that some clinics had in-house pharmacies to fill the prescriptions, which included such highly addictive substances as oxycodone and hydrocodone.

Boosted in part by strong new state laws forbidding such drug distribution systems, authorities have done a commendable job in launching the nationwide crackdown on pill mills and the doctors who profit from them. Even so, far more needs to be done in order to clamp down on this increasingly pervasive problem. Among my primary suggestions, which mirror those of many top officials including the nation's drug czar, Gil Kerlikowske:

- **Databases**: The various states need to jointly start and operate a database, in order to pinpoint and target any doctor who over-prescribes pain killers, and also to identify and target patients who seek excessive amounts of such prescriptions.

- **New Legislation**: The legislatures of some states including Florida should go ahead with plans already submitted by some lawmakers, requiring that any patient who receives such drugs first undergo examinations by doctors at pain clinics.

- **Increase Penalties**: Intensify and tighten the proverbial noose, making $10,000 fines and six-month suspensions mandatory for physicians found guilty of over-prescribing such medications.

- **Doctor Shopping**: Use the information from the database to prevent attempts by patients to obtain multiple prescriptions for pain medications in numerous states. Meantime, a handful of states already have programs to monitor such prescriptions, including Kentucky and Tennessee.

Despite these regulations already either proposed or suggested by various officials, our leaders need to do much more to clamp down on Big Pharma, which makes no significant effort whatsoever to limit these over-prescriptions. Instead of just blaming doctors and patients, authorities need to tighten their grips on the free-flowing and unchecked distribution of harmful pain killers to the pill mills.

Why Do Efforts Fail to Regulate the Flow of Pain Killers?

News reports indicate many doctors are willing to issue unnecessary pain killer prescriptions due to plain old-fashioned greed. This situation worsens when factoring in extreme problems for society and to the individuals involved.

Various publications claim that the abuse of prescription drugs— primarily pain killers—afflict at least 7 million people nationwide of age 12 and older. If true, this would make such addictions the third most widely abused drugs in the United States, behind alcohol and marijuana.

Greedy drug pushers and money-hungry doctors who issue too many pain killer prescriptions know that for just more than a few hundred bucks, patients at pill mills or who receive unnecessary prescriptions from standard physicians can get about 100 pills. Those same drugs obtained on the legitimate market are sometimes then sold by the gram, with a street value of about $5,400, experts say.
Besides ravaging the finances of entire families, prescription-level pain killer narcotics damage and permanently wreck the minds and bodies of those suffering the highest levels of abuse. Many of the most frequently abused drugs fall within the realm of high-level

analgesics at least to some degree, ranging from psychoactive drugs to performance enhancing narcotics.

Once again, keep in mind that substances in the psychoactive class alter everything from mood and levels of consciousness to behavior and even the ability to assimilate information. And, as you've already learned, drugs within the performance-enhancing class include highly dangerous anabolic steroids.

Taken individually or in mixtures of various substances, these many drugs slam deep into the lives and families of those who get hooked. Spouses and children of the primary drug abuser often suffer, especially when finances get depleted, the addict undergoes physical and mental deterioration, and relatives feel hopeless in efforts to save their loved ones from permanent physical and mental degradation.

Besides long-term heartlessness toward their relatives, many drug abusers commit robberies, burglaries and assaults in efforts to get money necessary to feed their habits.

Primarily for these reasons, we all need to remain cognizant of the potential extreme dangers of such drugs. When and if you legally take such substances under a physician's care, follow instructions carefully and strive from the start to avoid becoming addicted. And, if you, a loved one, friend or acquaintance shows early signs of such behavior, try to seek professional help as soon as possible.

Never Legalize Highly Powerful Pain Killers

Using arguments that I personally find bizarre and convoluted, some people proclaim that narcotics and especially pain killers should be legalized and made widely available. These individuals insist that our prisons are clogged with drug abusers and distributors, but that public resources would be better used in the rehabilitation process outside of penitentiaries.

Proponents of legalized substance abuse, such as the late "tune-in, turn-on, and drop-out" advocate Timothy Leary, have insisted that drugs of many kinds have proven relatively harmless when legally administered to entire societies. From this way of thinking, at least to a degree, the abuse of illegal substances has been equated to the prohibition era when the U.S. government outlawed the production, distribution and sale of alcohol.

Herein rests several extraordinary and pivotal questions: Would legalizing narcotics cut down on crime, abuse, excessive and extraordinarily high "street prices" for narcotics—while also alleviating prison overcrowding? Would legalizing the distribution and sale of extremely strong painkillers such as morphine, opium and heroin lessen the great potential harm posed by such substances on all of society? You be the judge.

Without question, these are pivotal dilemmas that will continue to face almost the entire world, especially as national, state, provincial and local governments struggle with increasingly problematic budget crises.

With luck, researchers will eventually develop a reliable,

indisputable and 100-percent effective non-addictive pain killer—
perhaps thanks largely to the Human Genome Project. For the time
being, however, the probability of whether scientists can develop
such a medication remains only a mere possibility.

When and if such advancement finally occurs, authorities
worldwide could then destroy all opium plants and other
substances. This would potentially eliminate at least a great
number of the many specific types of addictions to pain killers.

Yet, in the big scope of things, I find this situation almost
impossible. After all, why would pharmaceutical companies ever
entertain the very notion of cutting off a huge hunk of their own
stranglehold on the pernicious multi-billion-dollar mainstream
drug industry?

While society remains saddled with all these many dilemmas, at
least one thing remains certain. In all likelihood human beings
will continue to experience physical pains through the end of this
century and perhaps even for hundreds or thousands of years. For
as long as mankind thrives and prospers, people will continue to
suffer from these physical sensations.

To be sure, pain management is likely to continue evolving as
a unique and integral aspect of what some sociologists call the
"human experiment." As the many advancements and positive
developments in the ongoing battle against pain continues in the
coming decades, scientists and doctors should have plenty of good
news to announce.

PART TWO
Nature's Safe Pain Treatments

Chapter 8

Six Rungs on Everyone's Pain"Ladder"

Following a tradition or system first embraced by oncologists, many physicians use what is sometimes referred to as the "pain ladder." For the most part this process usually entails starting at the bottom of the proverbial ladder, initially prescribing low-dose or less addictive drugs with minimal side effects such as aspirin, or the equivalent of common over-the-counter drugs.

When and if a particular phase or step at this lower-rung fails to mask or eliminate pain, the physician might consider prescribing a stronger analgesic. The middle-rungs often involve weak or increasingly strong opiates, plus potential combinations of other drugs such as aspirin or over-the-counter products. At the top rung are the full-fledged opiate-class pharmaceuticals.

The ultimate objective is to prescribe super-strong and highly addictive opiates only when necessary. And conversely, as pain eventually lessens, an illness subsides or a wound heals, physicians can step down this proverbial pain ladder. This way doctors steadily begin administering the less potent medications.

Physicians and pharmaceutical companies often administer a combination of analgesics, depending on the specific severity of pain or the illness involved. For instance, remedies might include over-the-counter analgesics along with antihistamines to fight flu symptoms such as fever, muscle pains, a runny nose and watery eyes.

But many physicians warn any efforts to mix drugs should be done with extreme caution. According to a 2010 article in the *Australian Prescriber*, combining analgesics can sometimes generate confusion and result in accidental overdoses when using multiple drugs, some not necessary or not intended for the patient's specific symptoms.

In addition, rather than orally or via injection, some analgesics such as ibuprofen, capsaicin and diclofenac are administered as gels—rubbed onto the body's surface at the site of painful muscles or joints. Meantime, physicians sometimes inject steroids or the anesthetic Lidocaine into painful joints to generate long-term pain relief.

Adding to their many options, some doctors seeking to relieve or mask pain also administer anticholinergic agents, any substance that blocks neurotransmitters within the body's central nervous system. These range from Orphenadrin in treating painful muscle spasms to Cyclobenzaprine, a muscle relaxant medication.

Physicians and Patients Use a Popular Reference Book

The widely popular and highly respected "Physicians Desk Reference" serves as a bible or dictionary on a vast range of pain killers and medications for various illnesses. Commonly called "The PDR," this regularly updated book features a description of all primary, basic or advanced pain killers and other pharmaceutical products made by the major drug companies.

Available in bookstores, libraries and via Web connections to subscribers, the PDR serves as a valuable reference source for physicians, a wide range of medical professionals and by consumers curious about drugs they currently use or might get. Most descriptions feature images of the actual pills or products.

Certainly, this book for basic knowledge can help satisfy the curiosity of patients interested in inquiring about the many countless specific pain medications. However, you should remember that if and when using this publication, keep in mind that the most powerful pain medications used in the mainstream allopathic medical industry can only be issued by a licensed physicians. As always, I can't seem to stress enough that patients should never attempt to diagnose their own illnesses.

Despite what experts cite as the many advantages of the PDR, some patients remain cognizant that the publication lacks integral information on many of the basic natural substances often prescribed by homeopaths. The vast majority of the natural products that homeopaths recommend are not amassed, distributed or sold by the world's largest pharmaceutical companies.

Other critics of the PDR also complain that some listings on specific drugs are incomplete, or that data on numerous individual pharmaceuticals is sometimes listed before researchers have finished integral studies on new or developing medications. Adding heat to the issue, some observers contend that pharmaceutical companies often supply the PDR's producers with information that sometimes lacks details on potential negative side effects. In every yearly edition the PDR allows for "off-label" use of every drug listed.

From my view, for patients the PDR is best suited as a basic reference guide, in essence a dictionary for determining basic details on what they're either already taking or what a physician prescribes or recommends for them. As a patient, you should always feel free to ask your doctor or pharmacy professionals for the specifics on any drug you're taking such as recommended precautions such as whether to avoid meals or driving.

The Six 'Rungs' And How To Apply Them

There is virtually no specialty or sub-specialty of medicine or surgery that does not deal with pain in some form on an everyday basis. Even Psychiatry deals with emotional pain and the residual pain of post-traumatic stress disorder (PTSD).

Most doctors, but especially those in Anesthesiology, Neurology, Oncology, Neurosurgery, Orthopedic Surgery, Sports Medicine, Physical Medicine and Pain Medicine are familiar with the term "pain ladder". This, simply stated, means starting at the bottom rung of the ladder to determine which of the various prescription or non-prescription supplementations and/or treatments would be the best to treat the mildest forms of either acute or chronic pain, or discomfort, and then progressing up the ladder to achieve optimal control.

The first rung may in fact begin without the use of any over-the-counter supplements meant to be active in control of mild pain. These decisions are left up to the individual's caregiver, whether it be a doctor, nurse, physician's assistant or advanced practitioner of nursing. Most often this means prescribing any or all of the following substitutes for oral, topical, intramuscular, subcutaneous or intrathecal prescriptions. In no particular order, these include: Acupuncture, Pilates, Yoga, infrared saunas, plain/dry/or moist heat, thermal therapy (far infrared rays), biofeedback, physical therapy, aqua-therapy, chiropractic adjustments, hypnosis, or simple forms of exercise and stretching.

Any or all of the above would constitute likely candidates for the first rung of the ladder.

The next rung of the ladder (rung #2) usually contains a variety of over-the-counter topical agents, often referred to as "liniments" or "ointments", including the prescription drug "Lidoderm", which is a patch placed on the skin over the anatomical site of the muscular or skeletal pain.

These topical preparations may contain a form of aspirin called methyl salicylate. Other ingredients in these preparations may include chloroform or ethyl ether, Capsaicin, and mixtures of topical anesthetic agents.

Milder lotions for thermal and sunburns often contain aloe in various forms from the cactus plant. DMSO used as an ointment is popular in veterinary medicine but has also been used occasionally in mild cases of painful human musculoskeletal injuries or conditions.

I would also include on this rung of the pain ladder, the Homeopathic procedure called "neuro-therapy", in which a small #27-gauge or smaller needle in a 1.0 to 3.0 mL syringe is filled with a combination of a topical anesthetic (procaine) and vitamin B12. This mixture is injected intradermally, along acupuncture meridia or along cutaneous scars to alleviate minor pain complaints.

The next rung (#3) of the pain ladder would be the use of one or more supplements useful for chronic pain, preoperative pain, pregnancy, or just because the user does not want to suffer the side-effects of prescription drugs or risk addiction. These supplements are, for the most part, over-the-counter and do not have the usual side-effects of prescription drugs which can include a wide variety of unpleasant and troublesome symptoms, including: (1) Sedation; (2) constipation; (3) loss of appetite; (4) mental sluggishness; (5) retarded muscle reactions; and (6) rarely hallucinations or paranoia.

On this same rung I would include the popular combination of glucosamine - a sugar with an amine side chain - and chondroitin - a protein molecule. Both of these are precursors to the manufacturing of cartilage and are useful in osteoarthritis, rheumatoid arthritis, and post-traumatic arthritis.

A study by the National Institute of Health (N.I.H.) determined that the product glucosamine and chondroitin sulfate provided significant pain relief compared to a placebo. The side-effects of this combo are rare but can include gas, bloating and mild diarrhea.

On rung #3 I would also include SAMe - a sulfur-containing aminoacid that has been effective in treating minor joint pains and has a side-effect for providing relief for mild depressive illnesses, and for the neurologic symptoms of early Parkinson's disease. Like glucosamine-chondroitin, mild gastrointestinal side-effects such as gas, bloating and diarrhea, may be noticed but are usually insignificant.

Also, at this level of pain, Omega-3 fatty acids, which serve as anti-inflammatory agents, are useful adjuncts for treating mild forms of arthritis, musculoskeletal injuries, and post-traumatic painful injuries.

There are a number of miscellaneous prescription drugs which are useful for various types of pain, including migraine headaches, minor arthritic pains, musculoskeletal sports injuries or traumatic injuries, neuropathic pains, sympathetic dystrophies (i.e., Complex Regional Pain Syndrome (CRPS), formerly known as Reflex Sympathetic Dystrophy or RSD), phantom pains associated with amputations, and cluster headaches, just to name a few. Examples of these products include the following:

(1) Catapres - a prescription drug that is centrally active and is usually used as an antihypertensive agent can be used for treatment of CRPS and in various neuropathic painful conditions, such as postherpetic neuralgias.

(2) Dilantin - an anticonvulsant prescription medicine which can be useful for the treatment of refractory neuropathies.

(3) Botox (from the product botulism toxin) - a potent neurotoxin which when used in diluted doses can relieve stubborn migraine headaches.

(4) Mexitil - an antiarrhythmic prescription medication is used rarely to control chronic pain from various muscular disorders.

(5) Tambocor (a sister drug to Mexitil and also an antiarrhythmic)

- can also be useful for treating a wide variety of chronic pain disorders, including CRPS, post-chemotherapy neuropathies, and post-traumatic nerve injuries.

(6) Neurontin - another prescription drug which is useful to treat diabetic and postherpetic neuropathies, as well as neuropathic pains associated with various malignancies, i.e., lung cancer neuropathies.

(7) Direct injections into joints with local anesthetics, such as procaine, along with an accompanying steroid such as Kenalog are also effective for treating serious joint injuries, tendon and ligamentous injuries, as well as acute bursitis.

(8) The use of Indocin, a nonsteroidal anti-inflammatory agent, is useful for treatment of acute gouty arthritis as well as osteoarthritis, rheumatoid arthritis, and sports injuries accompanied by musculoskeletal pains.

Because Indocin is frequently a cause of gastritis or peptic ulcer disease, and as such it should be used cautiously and only for a short period of time (for example, two to four weeks maximum). Indocin is sometimes used with the addition of an over-the-counter anti-ulcer medication, such as Pepcid, Zantac or Tagamet.

(9) A number of vitamins often combined in a proprietary formula can also be included either individually or in combination for treatment of various minor pain conditions. These include vitamins B_6, B_{12}, and vitamin C. These vitamin supplements are most helpful for neuropathic pains, such as diabetic neuropathy, and postherpetic neuropathy.

(10) Alpha-Lipoic Acid (ALA) has also been shown in the Alternative Medicine literature to be a valuable adjunct in treating neuropathies similar to those responding to vitamins B_6 and B_{12}.

(11) Herbal products of various sources, either alone or in combination, can be of value for treatment of patients with mild to moderate pain, and these are appropriate to this rung of the ladder. This include:

A. Black Cohosh - This herbal product has been used to treat menstrual and menopausal-related pains, as well as minor arthritic conditions.

B. Cat's Claw, or so-called Una D' Gato has seen success in treating fibromyalgia pains and other mild musculoskeletal injuries.

C. Evening Primrose Oil (EPO) is a saturated fatty acid and has seen benefit in treating rheumatoid arthritis and osteoarthritis.

D. Arnica (mountain daisy) is a herbal product widely used in Homeopathy for treatment of sports injuries, fibromyalgia syndrome, and mild osteoarthritis symptoms.

E. Ginger - most noted for relieving nausea and vomiting, even post-chemotherapy nausea, has been of some benefit. However, it has also been shown to be effective in assisting treatment of the minor pains associated with osteoarthritis and post-traumatic arthritis.

F. Ginkgo biloba (Gingko) - an herbal product which helps with leg pains due to poor circulation (claudication), has also been seen benefit in multiple sclerosis-related leg cramps.

G. Tumeric (Curcumin), which can be used orally or topically, has been very popular in India for treatment of traumatic or post-surgical wound pain and mild arthritides.

H. St. John's Wort (hypericum), mostly known for its benefit for treatment in mild depression, has also shown positive activity in multiple sclerosis pains and neuropathic nerve pain injuries.

Other miscellaneous herbal preparations include the following, in no particular order:

A. Stinging nettle
B. Ledum (marsh tea)
C. Rhus-tox (poison ivy)
D. Ruta (rue)
E. Symphytum (comfrey)
F. Calendula (marigold)
G. Wild lettuce
H. Cayenne
I. White willow bark
J. Dogwood
K. Devil's Claw
L. Yucca
M. Feverfew
N. California poppy
O. Meadow Sweet
P. Boswilla
Q. Green tea extract
R. Bromelain
S. Chinese licorice
T. Black pepper extract
U. Jujube extract
V. Heartwood

There have also been a number of helpful minerals in relieving mild pains from arthritis and musculoskeletal injuries. These include magnesium, manganese, copper, zinc and selenium.

The 4th rung of the ladder begins with the mildest form of narcotic prescription drugs and also contains some of the few non-narcotic/non-steroidal anti-inflammatory drugs (NSAID's), some of which are still prescription drugs, however, many are obtainable over-the-counter at the present time. Some of the non-narcotic group of medications include:

A. Celebrex - useful in treating arthritis, both osteoarthritis and rheumatoid arthritis, but it has also been used as an adjuvant treatment for cancers, especially colorectal cancer.

B. Motrin - This NSAID is effective when given with many mild, moderate or heavy-duty narcotics, when used in between narcotic usage. For instance, a morphine tablet which is taken once every six hours, the Motrin could be used in between the six-hour dose on each occasion. It is available over-the-counter in a 200 mg. dose.

C. Ultram - a prescription non-narcotic analgesic, is usually given four times a day and is non-addicting.

The mildest narcotic pain medications include many of the following:

A. Codeine - either alone or in combination with aspirin or Tylenol.

B. Talwin - usually given from two to four times a day as a single agent.

C. Darvon - either alone or with Tylenol, usually taken every four to six hours.

D. Hydrocodone - either given alone in 5.0 mg, 7.5 mg or 10.0 mg doses every four to six hours as a single agent, or in combination with Tylenol.

It is important for patients to remember that 90 percent of all pain, even cancer-related pain, is treatable using the pain ladder, and before beginning the mild narcotic usage, the non-opiate alternatives and adjuvant therapies should also be tried to the maximum.

This rung #4 of the ladder is, in essence, the beginning of a
potential addictive risk to narcotic usage, but also contains
a number of frequent, unpleasant side-effects including: (1)
diminished appetite; (2) sedation; (3) chronic constipation; (4)
mental sluggishness and mild confusion; and (5) decreasing energy
and increasing fatigue.

When we talk about narcotics, it is often synonymous with the
use of pain pills for cancer as the brutal truth is that chronic pain
accompanies cancer in over 80 percent of patients. Even patients
with early cancer, up to 30 to 40 percent of them describe some
sort of pain.

Cancer pain may have many varieties depending upon the size and
location, and the rapidity of growth of the cancer itself. Pain is
usually steady, long-lasting, and as a rule not relieved by position,
eating or elimination. Pain has been described in various ways as
achy, throbbing, stabbing, or even burning. When cancer growths
are impinging upon nerve receptors in healthy tissues in solid
organs, on bony tissues and on blood vessels, any of these types
of pain may manifest. In fact, bone pain is the most common type
of pain seen in patients with advanced cancers, especially with
Stage IV cancers of the "big four" cancers - lung cancers, prostate
cancers, breast cancers, and colorectal cancers.

In addition to cancer pain itself, illnesses that frequently
accompany cancer, such as shingles, often produce severe pain
unilaterally, on one side or the other side of the body, and while the
rash itself accompanying shingles may only last two to four weeks,
the pain that it generates may last for months to years afterward.

For the short-acting, mild pain pills, if pain strikes primarily when you are up and around, doing exercises, walking, working at mild tasks or shopping, then the doctor may prescribe a short-acting, mild type of pain reliever.

On the other hand, if your pain is constant and present during resting hours as well as waking hours, then a long-acting pain reliever which needs to be taken only every eight to twelve hours may be preferable, or a pain patch which lasts for up to 72 hours may be the answer the doctor is looking for to solve the chronic pain problem.

From my personal experience of over 40 years practicing Medical Oncology and Integrative Oncology, I have found that prescription narcotic drug abuse is quite uncommon among cancer patients as they have a physical need for the medication and not a psychological need for the pain medication. However, if patients start taking pain medications more than the doctor has prescribed for, and if they do not stay faithful to a schedule, the possibility of addiction can increase, even if the patient goes into complete remission.

While it is true that most narcotic pain medications are opioids and are derived from several types of natural plants, there is an increasingly large number of synthetic versions which have been modified from their original opioid chemical structure.
It is true that hydrocodone (Vicodin) is a semi-synthetic opioid, similar in effects to morphine, and it is the most commonly prescribed medication in any category in the United States, and it is the most abused narcotic drug in the United States as of this writing.

Although opioids have little risk for serious health dangers or problems with organ dysfunction, such as effects on the heart, liver, kidneys, gastrointestinal or cardiopulmonary systems, they do have major side-effects including dizziness, drowsiness, headache, nervousness, tremor, anxiety, nausea, vomiting, constipation, itching, dry mouth or sweating. Many of these drugs also cause some hallucinosis or delusional behavior, and are frequently associated with some form of paranoia.

In regard to the fourth rung with the mildest form of narcotics, a physician will often go up a sub-ladder with the patient, using the lowest possible doses available as prescriptions, and then moving to the higher doses. In the case of Vicodin, one would start at a 5.0 mg dose, moving to a 7.5 mg dose, and then to a 10.0 mg dose. In addition to increasing the dosage, the physician could also increase the number of pills taken at any given time during the day, and then decrease the time interval between dosing. For instance, decreasing the Vicodin from every six hours' usage to every four hours' usage.

In short, there are many ways that the doctor has available to manipulate drug dosage in order to keep from going to the next higher level of efficacy or, in short, going up one more rung on the ladder.

Among the goals that doctors use to evaluate the effectiveness of a particular pain regimen, particularly a narcotic pain medication regimen, either with or without the use of adjuvant agents as mentioned above, would include the following:
1. Allowing a pain-free sleep interval of at least six hours per night.

2. Relief of resting pain.
3. Relief of lessening of pain with mild exercising or walking, such as gardening, housework or sedentary work in the office.

The #5 rung of the ladder involves the use of narcotics for moderate pain, not controlled by the fourth rung of the ladder in all of the many ways suggested above. Again, the use of adjuvant or helper drugs is paramount and always encouraged. The most common of these are Tylenol, Motrin, Aleve, Elavil and Ativan. In general, again it is important to exhaust all possibilities in the lower rungs before advancing to the next higher rung.

The major drugs for moderate pain treatment in this portion of the narcotic ladder would be the following:
1. Demerol
2. Percocet
3. Methadone
4. OxyContin
5. Duragesic patches
6. Sublingual Fentanyl Transmucosal Pain System

Again, like the milder forms of narcotics, every attempt is made to slowly increase the dose of the moderate analgesics one at a time, by starting at lower doses and then gradually working up the sub-ladders to the higher doses. Also, the number of pills can be increased so there can be two or three given at a time, or two or three patches at a time, and then the time interval between doses can be decreased as well. In addition to all of these factors, helper agents (as mentioned earlier) can all be used independently as adjuvant therapies to the narcotics to enhance the efficacy of the pain relief.

The next and highest rung of the ladder is the 6th rung. This rung contains the highest strength opioids, namely:
1. Dilaudid (hydromorphone)
2. Morphine Sulfate itself
3. MS-Contin

This level of the rungs is usually reserved for the most severely difficult to control cancer pains, postoperative pains, multiple traumatic injury pains, or fracture injury pains. Again, by increasing the doses of each potent narcotic, or by decreasing the time intervals of each narcotic, or going to a different form such as injectable, liquid form, subcutaneous pump, or rectal suppository, are all different modalities with varying degrees of success to achieve the ultimate results, and that is making the patient as pain-free as possible. Hospice care uses this rung.

The possibility of combining several rungs together has been used in the past, but it is always better to use one single agent and increasing the doses rather than to combine two or three different narcotics, which may all have additive side-effects and provide worsening side-effects and averse events for the patients themselves.

My Medical Clinic Attracts People
from Around the World

Many of them blessed with faith and filled with hope, each week people from around the world travel to my West Coast medical clinic. Members of my professional medical staff and my front-line employees tell me they're amazed by the continually growing number of patients. Many of these visitors first heard of me via word-of-mouth or various news media reports.

Others initially learned of my work to fight pain and disease through my various books, including one of my popular publications co-authored by media personality, actress and author Suzanne Somers. Needless to say, I feel humbled and honored every time various celebrities and many people worldwide eagerly endorse my clinics and various books.

From my view, the increasing popularity of my medical efforts stems from the methods I use to help fight pain plus the underlying ailments that ignite such symptoms. Besides the elimination of pain, patients visiting my clinic seek treatment for a wide variety of medical conditions ranging from cancer to immune disorders and general health issues.

Following 40 years in medical practice, I finally decided to generate this publication about physical pain at the urging of my many patients. Lots of these people can be seen in videos on my Website—DrForsythe.com—giving unsolicited personal heart-felt testimonials. The successful elimination of pain often hails as a primary topic.

I Get Pleasure from Helping Patients

At present, I'm one of only a handful of integrative medical oncologists in the United States and from throughout the world as well. An integrative medical oncologist is a fully licensed and certified medical professional who specializes in using standard allopathic medicines to treat cancer—plus non-traditional "natural" medicines such as herbs and vitamin treatments as well.

Like almost every other typical citizen, I become disturbed and highly concerned upon seeing other human beings suffer the ravages of crippling pain. During my first several decades in practice, I primarily used standard methods accepted by allopathic physicians when implementing cancer treatments. This typically meant the use of standard chemotherapy techniques, which invariably caused my patients to suffer extensive pain.

Besides the extensive decreases in body weight and the loss of hair, many cancer patients during the early part of my career died after courageously undergoing these horrific chemotherapy treatment regimens. Mirroring nationwide statistics at the time, only an extremely small percentage—slightly more than 2 percent—of my most advanced cancer patients survived for five years early in my career.

Determined to reverse these outcomes, during the mid- and late 1990s, I also became a certified and licensed homeopath. Such medical professionals specialize in natural treatments such as herbs, rather than standard drugs that often cause or fail to alleviate what I personally consider unnecessary and excessive pain—at least in some cases.

When integrating standard-practice medicines with natural holistic or homeopathic treatments, I found that the overall survival rates of my cancer patients dramatically increased. As the years progressed, I developed specific and specialized treatments to address pain, while also fine-tuning various regimens designed to target specific types of cancers and various other diseases. My program has been called the "Forsythe Immune Protocol" or "FIP," and encompasses all the modalities that I use.

Some Standard Physicians Disapprove of My Efforts

Amazingly, some standard allopathic physicians and neurologists disapprove of my professional efforts. Perhaps some of their displeasure stems from simple jealousy. For the most part, though, these doctors dislike the fact that I have been widely hailed as a maverick of sorts—someone willing to "rock the boat" for the betterment of patients.

All along, a key objective in my efforts has been the effective treatment of pain. Although many people describe my practice as highly successful in this regard, lots of standard-practice doctors have worked behind the scenes in hopes of discrediting my good name.

For the most part, these medical professionals embrace what they consider the only true and correct treatment regimens. These usually entail the distribution and use of standard drugs or "narcotics" produced by huge pharmaceutical companies, an overall industry nicknamed "Big Pharma."

The world's largest and richest drug companies have stabbed their proverbial hooks deep into the processes that run the American Medical Association and the federal Food and Drug Administration, also known as the FDA. Do you think these giant organizations truly care more about eliminating your pain and disease, or for making big bucks for themselves and for their shareholders?

From my perspective, greed plays an overriding and predominant role in the development of the various strategies and policies of these organizations. Most standard physicians follow and embrace this often-ineffective medical routine and they dislike the fact that I'm willing to stand tall and openly proclaim this fact. Ultimately, the big loser is you, the consumer, average patients who usually are given no other option than to consume unnecessary and potentially addictive drugs, at least in some cases.

Yes, now is the time for you to dig deeper into the underlying causes of pain, and to discover the various standard treatments that are likely to cause potentially harmful complications or unnecessary addictions. Just as important, you can look toward the path that I show, filled with natural remedies and treatments. Many of these strategies are specifically designed to target pain, in many cases eliminating such symptoms altogether.

Standard Physicians Tell You These Methods are "Far-Fetched"

Perhaps worried or fearful that the integrative medical practices such as mine will endanger their livelihoods, today's doctors within our mainstream American culture eagerly strive to label practitioners such as me as "quacks" or "mavericks."
Maybe this stems at least partly from the fact that pain and illness treatments that homeopaths recommend sometimes include non-traditional methods such as message, breathing and meditation exercises—or any of a wide variety of other methods seen as "off-the-wall" by mainstream physicians. Needless to say, today's "Big Pharma," the huge pharmaceutical conglomerates and standard-medicine doctors in the U.S. culture worry that they'll miss out on the big bucks if patients know they can go elsewhere.

The list of herbs, meditation styles and acupuncture treatments—all proven as consistently effective in the treatments of pain—is seemingly endless. And, of course, in the meantime many of the specific drugs and treatments embraced and commonly used in the mainstream U.S. medical industry also have proven effective as well. But many of these mainstream medications are ridden with severe and potentially fatal side effects.

While keeping the best, most effective medical methods from both cultures at the forefront, physicians such as me who fully understand, prescribe and embrace both systems have an opportunity to teach the general public. Personally, I feel obligated to educate patients worldwide that both medical systems have important roles in providing vital and necessary care to people who depend on our expertise.

Through the coming years, as society enjoys the continual new and improved advancements in medical technology, homeopaths and standard physicians must do more to appreciate and embrace each others' specific and general treatment methods.

From my view, in an ideal world, as we strive to battle the physical and emotional pains that plague our patients, physicians have an obligation to take essential, urgent and progressive strides in working for the betterment of the people we help. A key part of this process should entail the melding of the alternative homeopathic medicines and so-called mainstream medical practices.

Ideally, practitioners of these systems should meld their clinics, centralized in the same facilities. Such goals strike me and many other doctors as logical and even necessary for the betterment of patients. After all, standard allopathic physicians and homeopaths have already melded or integrated their practices in many other parts of the world including much of Europe and Asia.

Yet at least for the present, such overall efforts seem almost unmentionable within most of today's mainstream American culture. This leads me and the handful of other integrative physicians to openly pose such questions as, "If other areas of the world are benefiting patients by bringing together these medical systems, why should we be prevented from doing the same?"

Chapter 9

The Most Natural Pain Treatment of All

Perhaps the most grueling and painful physical activity that humans can engage in has to be the 'Ironman' competitions during which triathletes complete three continuous endurance events—running a marathon (26.2 miles), swimming 2.4 miles, and biking 112 miles. This event has been held annually in Hawaii since 1978.

To even finish the event despite the excruciating and unavoidable pain and discomfort, competitors must summon mental fortitude. Chrissie Wellington is a four-time World Ironman champion who achieved the distinction of winning her fourth title in 2011 despite having suffered serious injuries in a bad bike crash just two weeks before the race.

How does she do it? Grit, willpower, determination and mental strength, not sheer physical prowess, is how she explains her feats of endurance. "But how does one develop that strength?" she asks in her autobiography, *A Life Without Limits*. "Is it innate, or can it be learned? I believe it is the latter. We can train our brains to be as strong as our bodies."

She utilizes several techniques to help her keep exerting mind

over matter. She keeps a mantra or special song to repeat written on her water bottle and wristband to give herself an inspiring energy boost when she needs it. She memorizes a series of positive mental images and summons this imagery whenever the pain and exhaustion threatens to make her quit the race. The images can be of family or friends, or pleasant and soothing pastoral scenes. To create these images, she practices visualization exercises before each race, imagining the race and its successful completion.
She tries to stay focused during the race, breathing deeply and rhythmically to calm her mind.
Treating or preventing pain begins in the human mind. 'Mind over matter' effects constitute the most natural pain remedy we humans can call upon to enhance our experience of life.

Throughout recorded history in numerous societies, many ordinary people have literally walked on fire as if to prove that the power of their minds can prevent or ignore excruciating pain. Commonly referred to as "firewalkers," such people sometimes walk barefoot across extremely hot coals, stones or embers. These people somehow manage to avoid displaying or experiencing any sign of discomfort or injury.

These people attempt to convey a distinct message to the world, saying: "I'm powerful. My mind is everything, and the possibility of any pain at all means virtually nothing to me."

Some cultures use these occasions to test an individual's faith. Sure enough, within the psyche of humans, any perceived or actual victory over pain is often viewed as a great achievement worthy of eternal praise and of much well-deserved adulation.

Many religious faiths and diverse cultures have practiced this longstanding custom. Eastern Orthodox Christians, Taoists, Buddhists, and practitioners of certain African faiths have engaged in fire walking for thousands of years.

While any reasonable physician would never suggest or even recommend such behavior, firewalkers and people who advocate such activities refer to the process as healthy, or at least inspiring good health and personal growth. Some firewalkers work to strengthen or at least train their minds to focus on positive outcomes.

"A man is but a product of his thoughts, what he thinks he becomes," said Mohandas Gandhi, a pre-eminent advocate of civil rights and an ideological leader in the culture of India in the late 19th Century and early 20th Century.

People interested in the study, elimination and management of physical pain can easily find themselves mesmerized and intrigued by the many tales and historical accounts of such behavior. To most of us living in today's Western world, the mere notion of such a stroll can literally send shivers down our spines and make goose bumps erupt from head to toe.

Indeed, there is little denying that almost anyone who tries to walk on fire for the first time needs to employ what lay people often call a "leap of faith." Such attitudes might seem reasonable, because after all, since early childhood just about all of us are either taught to avoid extreme pain or we learn the hard way as toddlers, positioning ourselves to rarely ever repeat the same mistakes. Any small child who inadvertently puts his finger on a hot stove almost always learns to avoid repeating such behavior.

Besides expressions of religious or spiritual faith, some cultures use fire walking as an integral part of initiation processes, or even—as amazing as this might sound—as a form of spiritual or mental healing. The practice grew increasingly popular in the 1970s when advocates of "positive thinking" began embracing this process as a way for their students or practitioners to cross an essential "right of passage."

Attempts to "walk on fire" atop coals, blazing-hot rocks or other burning materials sometimes results in extensive injury, especially to anyone making such a stroll without expert guidance. Truly, in their effort to show their own strength of "mind over matter," some people go too far, too fast without first attempting to get sufficient information or without sufficient preparation and training.

When performed correctly, scientists say, pre-planned and well-choreographed fire walking efforts result in little or no injury whatsoever. Experts give much of the credit to the natural abilities of chosen materials to conduct or absorb the heat, rather than sending blazing hot temperatures outward into or through the walker's skin.

As Einstein eloquently stated, "everything is theoretically impossible, until it is done."

Use the Mind as a Powerful Weapon Against Pain

When treating pain, we should remain cognizant that the great power of our minds, and of our individual personal belief systems are formidable. Many important or famous events throughout history tell us that some people have used the strength of their minds to literally ignore or persevere despite potentially excruciating or debilitating physical pain.

Anyone suffering from extreme pain today can take at least some comfort in knowing that many people have survived severe discomforts before returning to good health.

On Dec. 7, 2007, a 37-year-old window washer plummeted 47 stories on a scaffolding that became disengaged from a Manhattan skyscraper. According to news accounts, Alcides Moreno suffered from many broken bones throughout his entire body. Thanks to modern medical techniques physicians strived to control Moreno's pain, while successfully performing multiple surgeries.

Moreno's brother Edgar had died in the same accident. Thanks largely to his own determination coupled with the moral and professional support of his surviving family members and physicians, Alcides Moreno was soon on track for a full recovery. While many people worldwide considered Moreno's recovery as miraculous, his case also serves as a prime example of how patients and physicians can successfully work together to overcome the ravages of extreme pain, injuries or disease.

Any time a physician tells you to "get your affairs in order" because there is no hope of eliminating your physical pain, and that same medical professional also tells you that there is "no hope of survival," you should immediately find a new doctor.

Have Faith That You Can Beat Pain

For countless generations people from many cultures have embraced that age-old adage proclaiming that "faith can move mountains."

As a practicing oncologist, homeopath and a Christian, I have personally witnessed many instances where people have used their personal, spiritual and religious faith in beating the so-called odds. At least to some degree what the masters say essentially holds true, that each of us ultimately becomes what we think we are.

If you consider yourself as whipped, a loser and beaten down forever by pain, you likely will evolve into just such a person. Conversely, those of us who strive to put ourselves in a positive, peaceful and pain-free light often find ourselves in just such a position.

As the writer Patrick Overton once proclaimed, "When you have come to the edge of all light that you know and are about to drop off into the darkness of the unknown, faith is knowing one of two things will happen—there will be something solid to stand on, or you will be taught to fly."

Certainly faith remains an essential medicine for patients suffering from pain, perhaps just as important in many cases as the various pharmaceuticals and treatments that a physician might prescribe. To ignore any possibility of embracing faith is essentially the equivalent of slapping the possibility of potential recovery clean across the face.

"You block your dream when you allow your fear to grow bigger than your faith," said Mary Manin Morrissey, a minister in Oregon.

Filled with faith that they can whip the ravages of pain and illness, every year more than 5 million people hailed as pilgrims visit the small town of Lourdes, France—which has a population of only 15,000. There, the faithful visit the Sanctuary of Our Lady of Lourdes, where believers say that Mary the Mother of Jesus made numerous visits in 1858 to Saint Marie Bernarde-Soubirous when she was only 14 years old.

The Roman Catholic Church has officially recorded at least 67 miraculous healings generated by the water at the sanctuary. Officials who reviewed these cases insisted that they were unable to find any psychological or physical reason for why these cures occurred, other than to conclude that "miracles" had happened.

For believers and perhaps some non-believers alike, this shrine has generated much curiosity and thereby has inspired significant hope. From my personal view, the vast majority of human beings desperately want to believe in something significant. People yearn to know and to realize within their hearts and deep inside their souls that their physical and emotional pains can and will be permanently eradicated.

Some scientists insist the water of Lourdes lacks any medicinal qualities whatsoever. And, at least judging by some widespread published accounts, the water also lacks any provable curing powers. Even so, those who believe in the miracles that occurred at the sanctuary still consider the water as an enduring symbol of faith and hope.

Certainly, any attempt to rob people of their faith in cures and that pain can be eliminated would be worse—at least in a sense—than trying to steal millions of dollars in gold from them. To the interminable human spirit, hope and faith are more precious than all the riches that our physical world could possibly provide.

"Be not afraid of life," said James Truslow Adams, a 20th Century American writer and historian. "Believe that life is worth living, and your belief will help create the fact."

Embrace and Benefit from the Tremendous Power of Prayer

Each day while alone in my office, and on Sundays at church services, I quietly pray for the physical recovery of my patients and for their individual improvements against the ravages of pain.

Like millions of other Americans, I strongly believe in the awesome power of prayer. According to an article in *USA Today*, a whopping 83 percent of people responding to a survey said they believe that God answers our prayers. And, just as impressive, 92 percent of those surveyed indicate they believe there is a God.

According to the Pew Research Center's Forum on Religion and Public Life, a 2007 survey indicated that six out of 10 Americans reported that they pray every day.

The same U.S. Religious Landscape Survey indicated differences in the frequency of prayer, the amount of such activities conducted by people from various religions, and the income, age and gender of the faithful. Among the survey's findings:

- **Age groups:** A total 68 percent of people older than age 65 pray every day. That's the highest percentage of any age group surveyed, according to a forum press release. The smallest percentage from any surveyed age group that prays daily is from ages 18-25 at 48 percent; the percentage totals steadily increase with each progressively older age group, before cresting at the age 65 and above bracket.

- **Gender:** Sixty-six percent of females pray daily, compared to only 49 percent of males

- **Income levels:** Sixty-four percent of lower-income individuals earning less than $30,000 yearly indicate they pray daily, compared to only 48 percent of people who earn more than $100,000.

Throughout my medical career, I have seen many cases that seemed to show that the power of prayer generates undeniably positive results that some people would consider "miracles." Many of these improvements in the various medical conditions of these individuals might have resulted from the power of the mind, specific medical treatments, or perhaps even instances of unexpected natural recovery.

As a physician, I concentrate on scientific- and natural-related treatments rather than serving as a spiritual or religious advisor. Nonetheless, to any patient who happens to ask, I give my honest belief that prayer can and does serve as a significant and powerful force.

Data Shows the Mega-Powerful Force of Prayer

During the past several hundred years, there have been numerous well-documented and verified cases of people who have been condemned to die—only to eventually survive the execution process, possibly thanks at least in part to the tremendous power of prayer.

As you can very well imagine, each of these surviving individuals endured intense physical and emotional pain during the execution process. But in each of these cases, including some that involved the awesome power of prayer, the condemned people survived and then were allowed to live.

Without any publicity whatsoever, patients suffering from usually fatal levels of illness and extreme pain survive, literally beating the odds. At emergency rooms, patient rooms and in doctor's offices nationwide, some patients get the much-awaited joyous news that their diseases have gone into remission and their pain subsides. The vast majority of these occurrences get little or no publicity.

Indeed, miracles are occurring every day, seemingly all around us and yet we rarely ever realize all this is happening. Those of us within the medical profession who serve as close insiders to individual cases take great pride when such instances occur.

Unlike most condemned people who know they will die after a last-possible appeal gets denied, for many standard patients there is almost always at least some degree of hope—for as long as they remain alive, and for as long as they feel the pain.

Certainly, those of us in the medical profession who deal with daily life-and-death decisions often notice that this longtime saying remains true—"Man can live about 40 days without food, about three days without water, about eight minutes without air, but only for one minute without hope."

Humor Can Be A Potent Mind Tool

Throughout my many years as a physician, I have personally witnessed countless instances where people bravely faced horrific pain—often resorting to humor as a powerful weapon to help alleviate their mental and physical anguish.

By their very nature, the vast majority of people are "fighters" who yearn to win and to persevere through the midst of real or perceived hardships. Yes, Mother Nature commands that we struggle to remain alive and stay vibrant for as long as possible. And, for the most part, humor invariably plays an integral role in helping to enable at least some of us to cope with these struggles.

In the 1999 comic film "Patch Adams," superstar Robin Williams played a widely acclaimed real-life American physician, Hunter Doherty "Patch" Adams. Also an active author and social activist, Adams organized volunteers who traveled the world—dressed as clowns for entertaining patients, orphans and many other people.

Although Adams has been quoted as criticizing the film for portraying him as merely a funny doctor, there is no denying that humor and basic entertainment such as the shows he organized can go a long way toward helping people alleviate, ignore, or cope with pain—while also encouraging patients to take the path toward eventual recovery.

Fully cognizant of the need to keep humor as an essential ingredient toward recovery, my professional medical and office staff maintains video tapes and discs of movies including many popular comedies. While many of my patients receive intravenous treatments such as certain chemotherapies or immune boosters, they often eagerly seize the opportunity to watch the films.

Silent film star Harold Lloyd made significant strides in enabling people to laugh at extremely painful situations, even suffering a horrendous real-life hand injury during the 1919 filming of "Haunted Spooks"—losing a thumb and index finger in a bomb blast. The injury forced Lloyd to wear a prosthetic glove in subsequent films, including "Safety Last" in 1923 where his character dangles from the bending hands of a clock near the top of a skyscraper. Nervous but excited audiences roared in laughter.

Silent film star Charlie Chaplain also delighted fans in classic films such as "The Gold Rush" in 1925, where his beloved "Tramp" character dangles from a cabin at the precipice of a cliff in the Klondike, battles an escaped fugitive, and carves a nail-lined boot in hopes of enjoying a tasty meal.

The reasons why people often laugh hysterically at potentially painful situations may stem at least in part from the intensity of emotions we all instinctively know that such sensations often elicit. And, of course, the potential for great humor often seems to intensify when the danger threatens other people rather than us—

particularly to our perceived enemies or to individuals that we care little or nothing about.

Although failing to perform well at the box office, the Marx Brothers' 1933 anarchic film "Duck Soup" is now considered among history's greatest comedy movies as listed by the American Film Institute. Groucho Marx portrays Rufus T. Firefly, a character some observers say seemed loosely modeled after the Italian fascist Benito Mussolini—who actually ended up banning the film in that nation. The plot ridicules the absurdity of war and its resulting pain, death, injuries and destruction.

After starting their own successful act on Vaudeville, The Three Stooges spread their slapstick comedy worldwide in films distributed worldwide. Their comedy brand fit the mold of slapstick, where exaggerated violence greatly exceeded what most people would consider common sense. Their characters would go overboard, such as hitting each other over the head with hammers or throwing their adversaries or each other to the floor.

Use Slapstick Humor to Battle our Own Actual Pains

Historians tell us that the use of slapstick humor prevailed in many cultures through Europe and eventually the Americas beginning as far back as the Renaissance and even the Middle Ages. Some history buffs even argue that slapstick or dark humor sometimes even emerged as a key factor in Greek and Roman stage productions thousands of years ago. Today, while remaining fully cognizant that slapstick humor is pure farce, people suffering from severe pain can face their afflictions head-on—perhaps even erupting in a healthy laugh at their own current predicaments.

Even the great, unsurpassable bard Shakespeare in the late 1500s and early 1600s penned gripping, uproarious comedies that featured chase scenes with painful consequences and beatings. Perhaps the most notable among them in terms of slapstick, puns and mistaken identity was among his first works, "The Comedy of Errors." The plot even delves into such normally delicate topics as demonic possession, theft and even infidelity.

Some noted thespians even go so far as to say that in creating this production, Shakespeare used as his primary models two plays written in the second century before Christ by Titus Maccius Plautus. These ancient works marked the early beginnings of the slapstick genre, which gained widespread popularity in the American culture in the 1900s thanks largely to entertainment by such greats as Laurel and Hardy, and the Keystone Kops.

At the height of their own real-life discomforts, many people might consider the very idea of laughing at pain as unthinkable or perhaps even offensive. The paradoxical nature of such dueling mental motivations and opposite perspectives could very well confuse even the most seasoned practitioners of psychiatric medicine. Nonetheless, perhaps because human nature makes many of us want to laugh at pain, slapstick-style entertainment also blossomed into the arena of animated films.

Medical Science Studies Affirm Humor's Role

Humor and laughter's role in reducing pain and relieving symptoms associated with other ailments is well documented in the medical science literature. Physiologically it's a result of various pain reliever hormones being released when laughter occurs.

Here are just a few examples from hundred of studies showing how humor therapy works in practice:

"Humor therapy: relieving chronic pain and enhancing happiness for older adults." This June 2010 study in the *Journal of Aging Research* placed 36 people in a nursing home into an 8-week humor therapy program; 34 other people were in the control group not offered the program. The study authors concluded: "upon completion of the humor therapy program, there were significant decreases in pain and significant increases in happiness and life satisfaction for the experimental group, but not for the control group. The use of humor therapy appears to be an effective nonpharmacological intervention."

"Laughter, humor and pain perception in children: a pilot study." In this June 2009 study published in the *Evidence Based Complementary & Alternative Medicine* journal, a group of 18 children aged 7-16 years watched humorous videos before, during and after a standardized pain task. Pain severity ratings and pain tolerances were recorded. These UCLA researchers found that "the group demonstrated significantly greater pain tolerance while viewing funny videos."

"Humor as a cognitive technique for increasing pain tolerance." This November 1995 study in the journal, *Pain,* used four groups of people with 20 subjects in each. One group was shown a humorous film, the second a repulsive film, the third a neutral film, and the fourth group no film at all. Pain tolerances were tested using cold pressor stimulation. Both the humor and repulsive groups "showed a significant increase in pain tolerance as compared to the other groups."

James W. Forsythe, M.D., H.M.D.

Pets Also Can Play an Integral Role in Fighting Pain

Seasoned physicians and medical professionals from many
specialties have learned the increasing importance that pets can
play in helping us to alleviate pain or physical discomforts. Widely
respected and much-needed organizations such as Therapy Dogs
United have brought a positive impact to the lives of patients
in hospitals and individuals as they undergo essential physical
therapies. Medical studies have affirmed the important role that
pets can play in pain relief and illness recovery.

With increased frequency in recent years, hospitals and other
important medical facilities nationwide have accepted the vital
services of such volunteers. Trained or obedient dogs and cats
sometimes serve essential roles in what medial professionals call
animal-assisted therapy.

The primary objectives of such pet owners who volunteer their
time and energy are to assist patients in improving their cognitive
skills, social interactions, physical abilities and emotional well
being. Significant improvement in any or all these areas can go a
long way in helping to eliminate both physical and emotional pain.

Many such programs require that before being accepted the pets
must undergo rigorous veterinary examinations to help ensure the
animals are healthy enough for such activities, while also avoiding
the likelihood of spreading diseases.

Besides dogs and cats, according to a variety of published accounts
the various species recruited to assist in such efforts range from
elephants and llamas to lizards and rabbits.

Natural Painkillers

Every day, nationwide and around the world volunteers bring their animals to hospitals, medical clinics and physical therapy facilities for interaction with human patients.

Besides helping patients improve their abilities to move about freely, a process that medical experts call "motor skills," via animal-assisted therapy some patients also can enjoy improvements in their abilities to stand or to use mobility devices like wheelchairs.

Just as impressive, according to some research this process also sometimes goes a long way toward enabling patients to improve their self-esteem, while helping to reduce anxiety and loneliness. All along, some patients even re-learn the ability to trust.

Although some observers have called such therapies nothing more than a "dangerous fad," many medical professionals ardently believe such efforts provide essential value in the process of striving for physical and mental improvements.

Whether this process inspires or motivates participation in group activities, and improves interactions with others apparently remain questions for continued study. All along, many of those who participate in such activities insist the process has definite value.

According to one age-old saying about pets, "One reason a dog can be such a comfort when you're feeling blue is that he doesn't try to find out why." Those who embrace and encourage animal-assisted therapies encourage such observations.

"Animals are such agreeable friends," said Mary Anne Evans,

the 19th Century English novelist who wrote under the pen name George Eliot. "They ask no questions; they pass no criticisms."

Many advocates of animal-assisted therapies insist the process has an important and vibrant history. According to some published accounts, a U.S. Army soldier, Corporal William Wynne, was often visited by a Yorkshire terrier, "Smoky," while the man recovered from at a hospital in the Philippines during World War II.

Dr. Charles Mayo, namesake of the internationally acclaimed Mayo Clinic in Rochester, Minn., began taking Smoky on his rounds after the dog became increasingly popular among patients in the Philippines hospital. The dog emerged as a hit among patients and staffers, motivating them to continue using the pet in the therapy process for a 12-year period through the war and afterward.

Advocates using animals such as Smoky insisted that these visits helped reduce stress experienced by individual patients. As Doctor Mayo observed, "worry affects the circulation, the heart, the glands, the whole nervous system, and profoundly affects heart action."

Medical professionals in other parts of the globe also independently recognized the many benefits generated by visits from animals. In England, registered nurse Elaine Smith noticed improvements in patients after visits from a chaplain accompanied by his golden retriever. Inspired by these improvements, Smith returned to the United States, where she launched programs for training dogs for such visits. Now these 'Thera-pet" programs can be found in hospitals and nursing homes nationwide.

Chapter 10

Numerous 'Alternative' Medicines Battle Pain

Standard or mainstream physicians often frown upon various other alternative medicines. For thousands of years some of these traditional systems have proven effective in eliminating pain or removing the underlying conditions that cause physical discomfort, though many standard-practice doctors continue to believe that at least some, or perhaps all, alternative medicines lack any credible scientific or credible basis.

There is a myth that such treatments aren't based on credible results from evidence-based research. That simply isn't true. Countless patients worldwide also seem to feel otherwise, seeking out these treatments and often returning for follow-up checkups, treatments, herbs or therapy sessions.

Among just some of the many widely recognized alternative medical practices, listed here in alphabetical order:

- **Acupuncture**: Often in an effort to relieve pain, acupuncturists follow the ancient Chinese-based tradition and method of inserting and manipulating needles into specific regions of a patient's body. It is often effectively used in anesthesia. Besides pain relief, acupuncture strives to treat or prevent disease, in addition to the use as a therapy or to strive for good overall health. The methods and concepts embraced by acupuncturists often differ from the scientific-based strategies and diagnosis methods accepted by traditional doctors. Acupuncture emerged in ancient times, thousands of years before the advent of cellular theory, complex discoveries in biology and integral research into the human anatomy. Even after such scientific medical advances, many patients worldwide have sworn to what they call the great and reliable effectiveness of acupuncture. Also, acupuncture points are directly related to internal organ systems.

- **Biofeedback**: Modern-day science-based devices are attached to patients, who can then continuously monitor their own vital signs—everything from the heart rate and breathing rates to muscle tension, brainwaves and skin temperature. According to some published reports, biofeedback has proven effective in treating headaches and migraines as patients use the monitors while teaching themselves to relax, breathe slowly and to control their own sensations of pain.

- **Chiropractic Medicine**: Although labeled as "quackery" by some standard-practice doctors, this longtime and widely accepted branch of medicine has been hailed by many patients as effective in fighting severe pain such as backaches or joint aches. Following extensive education in

their crafts, doctors of chiropractic excel in diagnosing and
treating problems with the body's musculoskeletal system,
particularly the spine. Such professionals realize that the
spine plays an integral role in the body's nervous system,
particularly the integral and highly complex natural system
of experiencing pain. Some scientists label chiropractic
as an alternative or "complimentary" branch of medicine,
separate but potentially related to so-called primary care
physicians. When viewed in this regard, chiropractors
practice falls within a medical specialty like dentists or
podiatrists. Some chiropractors specialize primarily in
adjustments of the spine, while others concentrate on
that as well while also seeking to mix a variety of other
treatments such as herbal supplements or homeopathy.

To illustrate the potential value of chiropractic medicine
in treating pain, I want to share a story told by a
collaborator of mine, Randall Fitzgerald, in his 2006
book, *The Hundred Year Lie: How Food and Medicine
Are Destroying Your Health.* Fitzgerald described what
happened in the wake of a nasty fall he experienced
that injured the right side of his lower back: "Friends
rushed me to the emergency room of a hospital, where
I was hooked up to an intravenous morphine drip. The
morphine barely dulled my sensation of pain. X-rays for
broken bones were negative, and an attending physician
speculated that the fall had bruised one of my kidneys. He
wrote me a prescription for a strong narcotic painkiller
and sent me home with the confession, 'there is nothing
else that can be done for you.' As I walked in agonizing
pain to a neighborhood pharmacy {to fill the painkiller

prescription} I happened to pass by a chiropractic clinic. Though I had no reason to believe that a chiropractor could provide relief, my intuition urged me to at least inquire. A middle-aged chiropractor tended to me immediately and applied a heat compress to my lower back, followed by an ultrasound treatment. She then spent ten minutes doing deep tissue massage on the affected area. She explained how these manipulations combined with heat and sound –a synergistic effect—would help to restore the internal alignment of my kidney. Her technique worked like magic. I got off the table and my pain was instantly and completely gone, and it never returned."

- **Herbalism**: This specialty concentrates on a vast array of natural-grown plants and herbs that are extracts from plants. Also, some products or substances prescribed by herbalists include substances derived from animals or insects, such as bee venom or specific types of fungus. The many herbs and plant derivatives for fighting pain include meadowsweet, a perennial herb found naturally in Asia and Europe; this has salicylic acid—heralded for its ability to fight pain, reduce fever and relieve inflammation. Other natural pain relievers include plants found on Caribbean and Pacific islands, and a perennial flowering plant found in North America, Asia and Europe, "stinging nettle." More than 120 plants or herbs used in herbalism also are used in making drugs produced by Big Pharma, including some pain killers.

- **Lamaze**: This is among numerous natural childbirth techniques that teach women various methods of coping with extreme pain during labor—without resorting to traditional standard-medicine drugs to relieve pain. Lamaze is among natural birthing systems that some critics claim lacks any evidence-based proof that it works as an effective medical therapy. Nonetheless, many Lamaze proponents embrace and encourage this method, which entails everything from learning to breathe through the pain to massage and spontaneous pushing. Proponents of natural childbirth methods such as Lamaze proclaim this process hails as the healthy and much-preferred alternative to mainstream medical techniques. Many women who chose to give birth naturally fear that local anesthetics sometimes used by traditional mainstream physicians might pose potential harm to themselves or to their babies. Proponents of natural childbirth argue that women are biologically capable of giving birth without medical assistance.

- **Naturopathy**: Sometimes called naturopathic medicine, these treatments appreciate and recognize that the body possesses an innate ability for self-healing. Practitioners of naturopathy strive to minimize surgeries, while concentrating on a whole-body or "holistic" approach dealing with everything from the patient's mental, physical, bodily and mental conditions, perspectives or environments. Patients often are instructed to undergo a wide range of medicines and lifestyle choices, which can include a variety of exercises, herbs, nutritional objectives, stress reduction methods and acupuncture. Some professional practitioners of naturopathy employ a degree of traditional medicine in their overall approach to fighting pain, while others prefer to employ more alternative strategies such as those often used by homeopaths.

Besides these systems along with homeopathy and ancient Chinese medicine, people worldwide seek help from pain from a vast range of other alternative medicines. These include traditional therapies, plus medical disciplines from specific cultures or nations such as Tibet and Mongolia.

Literally hundreds of alternative medicine structures or philosophies still exist, such as intentional fasting, faith healing, using magnets for therapy, and countless others that I would rarely if ever recommend. Nonetheless, an age-old American proverb proclaims that "variety is the spice of life." Such zest and vibrancy within our mainstream medical culture is needed to give everyone a pathway to getting much-needed relief from pain. For those seeking any potential alternative medicine to relieve pain, I recommend that the person conduct extensive research before seeking such options.

Homeopathic Pain Therapies Prove Effective

Depending on individual conditions, circumstances and remedies, some natural homeopathic pain remedies are just as effective as expensive pills from Big Pharma.

When I make such irrefutable and well-documented assertions, many physicians and other professionals from standard-practice medicines begin to scoff and whine. Undoubtedly, many standard allopathic doctors fear that natural remedies will endanger their livelihoods. When this happens, are such physicians working in the best interest of patients, or primarily for the doctors' own financial gain?

Some researchers, scientists and standard-medicine doctors might tell you that "homeopathic medicines are only as good as a placebo." These whiners also sometimes proclaim that homeopathic substances lack the "pharmacology" or potency of pharmaceuticals made by the huge drug companies—some costing many dollars per pill.

Yet, I easily could find myself asking such complainers, "Why do you consider the much more costly drug more effective? Could your perception stem from the fact that Big Pharma pills are much more expensive than natural remedies?"

Topping this off, as a highly experienced physician now entering my fifth decade as a practicing physician and now as a registered homeopathic doctor as well, I have witnessed many instances where natural substances worked effectively on pain. This serves as a promising observation, especially because overall the dangerous drugs made by Big Pharma generate far more serious potential side effects.

In some instances the best treatments stem from the remedies embraced or recommended by standard medicines and Big Pharma. Even so, from my perspective common sense dictates that physicians should at least consider the potential remedies proposed by homeopathy, depending on the specific case and the symptoms involved.

Homeopaths choose from a wide range of potential substances for specific ailments, including the alleviation of pain. The many hundreds of options range from various combinations of salts, snake venoms, and thyroid hormone extracts. Some options also include various substances derived from living organisms that are deemed healthy.

Within this branch of medicine, such substances are often referred to as "remedies," although this term should never imply a guaranteed cure or a lessening of symptoms. Meantime, all practicing homeopaths recommend variations of exercise, a healthy diet and good physical hygiene such as cleanliness.

In preparing remedies issued by homeopaths, specific substances often are mixed or diluted with alcohol or distilled water. Some observers or critics point out that the mixing of various substances—sometimes intended for pain—might result in toxic reactions. From my perspective, this is among primary reasons why patients seeking homeopathic treatments should seek the services of only a licensed, highly trained homeopath.

Familiarize Yourself with Top Homeopathic Pain Medicines

While remembering that patients should never attempt to diagnose their own ailments, everyone should feel free to become familiar with some of the top pain-relief remedies used by homeopaths. Among the most common:

- **Arnica**: Some homeopaths insist this substance often emerges as highly effective in battling the excruciating pains and symptoms of arthritis. Technicians generate "arnica" into an herb, derived from a yellow flower that grows at high elevations in Europe. Patients using arnica usually apply this on the skin in the form of a gel, or orally.

- **Curcumin**: From the perspective of homeopaths, this helps lessen or prevent painful swelling. The body usually absorbs curcumin better when taken orally as a capsule. Sometimes called "turmeric," curcumin is also used as an anti-inflammatory in battling the potentially crippling symptoms of arthritis. Some patients prefer this to standard medicines for treatments to painful conditions like hemorrhoids.

- **Devil's claw**: People with pre-existing stomach problems should avoid this often-powerful homeopathic remedy, derived from a fruit that grows in South Africa and often found effective in treatments for everything from backaches to arthritis.

- **Feverfew**: Homeopaths use this flowering plant prevalent across North America, Europe and the Mediterranean to generate a medicinal herb—often deemed helpful in generating relief from the pain of headaches and arthritis.

- **Frankincense**: Perhaps best known worldwide as one of the gifts the three wise kings brought the Infant Jesus along with gold and myrrh, this aromatic resin from the hardy boswellia trees in Armenia is often used in perfumes and even incense. And, besides its use in religious rites, frankincense can be eaten in pure form—a treatment used for hundreds of years for arthritic pain and minor injuries. Some researchers indicate they're studying the possible effects of frankincense on numerous specific painful afflictions, including ulcerative colitis and Crohn's Disease, which inflames the intestines.

Varying homeopathic medicines or generalized treatments within this realm have been used for thousands of years, at least according to some published reports. In the late 1700s and early 1800s, the German physician Samuel Hahnemann played an integral role in generating what many people today call "alternative medicine." Even then Hahnemann, the "father of homeopathy," believed that the so-called traditional medicines of his era did "more harm than good."

Exercise or Physical Therapy Also Plays a Vital Role

Besides good nutrition, exercise and the administering of specific drugs or remedies, the process of physical therapy plays a vital and essential role in the fight against pain. Those who undergo physical therapies range from people injured in accidents to those who suffered strokes, severe illness or chronic ailments.

Conducted by certified physical therapists, this primary health care process strives to enable people to regain or retain their abilities to move their bodies in a natural, functional way. Physical therapy can help improve posture and also boost overall health, thereby potentially lessening or eliminating pain.

Patients who undergo physical therapy often are encouraged to make such efforts a lifelong process. This stems largely from a continual need to remain vigilant at striving to move, walk or pick up objects in natural ways, even amid persistent and chronic ailments, advanced age, or certain irreversible after-effects from injuries.

The process of re-learning to move certain ways or improving

muscular functions via physical therapy can help improve
bodily functions and the psyche as well. Such improvements
sometimes generate more positive attitudes in patients, sparking
or re-energizing motivations that enable them to battle their own
physical discomforts.

Many certified and much-respected specialties of physical therapy
target everything from neurology and pediatrics to centers for
cardiopulmonary patients and facilities focusing on the unique
needs of senior citizens.

Starting with hydrotherapy, massage and manual therapy nearly
500 years before Christ, the earliest physicians of the Greek culture
including Hippocrates reportedly began to recognize the value
of continually attempting to resume body movements. Physical
therapies blossomed in the late 1800s in Britain. The process
soon spread to America, where remedial exercise increased as an
important aspect of such treatments.

This field of medicine surged amid the polio outbreak of 1916,
followed soon afterward by World War I when physicians began
recruiting nurses to assist wounded soldiers in active efforts to
regain their abilities to move in natural ways.

Today, the many neurological disorders or functions targeted by
specific physical therapies include such painful or debilitating
conditions as stroke, Parkinson's Disease, brain injuries, cerebral
palsy, and joint replacements such as the hip.

Anyone now fighting painful conditions while suffering from
physical disabilities should ask a certified medical professional

whether physical therapy might help eliminate pain. Some medical insurance plans cover most costs for such treatments.

"Depending on your individual circumstance, physical therapy might go a long way in enabling you to battle pain," I tell some patients, especially those who inquire. "The best way to determine that possibility is to first conduct a complete diagnosis, and then we'll take it from there."

Needless to say, physical exercise boosts the immune system while improving bodily functions such as muscular tone and bone strength. These functions can go a long way toward preventing or lessening the probability of painful conditions. Meantime, these overall improvements in the patient's ability to move or lift objects can enable the individual to recover more rapidly from illness or injury, particularly if extensive and regular exercise begins well beforehand.

Athletic coaches and military generals have known for many generations that their athletes or soldiers who have well-conditioned bodies have decreased chances of injuries and an improved likelihood of quick recoveries if physical problems should occur.

Besides honing their mental skills and fine-tuning the abilities to conform to rules or necessary skill-sets, well-conditioned soldiers and athletes reportedly have faster and better mental reactions in challenging and potentially dangerous situations. Such high-level mental functioning can increase the person's ability to escape painful results.

In both military and sports settings, well conditioned bodies also can increase the likelihood of victory for the entire team. While going a long way to battle or prevent potentially painful outcomes, this philosophy of excellent physical conditioning often spills over into the important professions of firefighters, police officers and prison personnel.

Two Pain Fighting Exercise Programs

Using six separate 30-second therapeutic movements, Dr. Joseph Weisberg presents a program in his 2005 book, *3 Minutes to a Pain-Free Life,* to strengthen the musculoskeletal system for pain prevention. It's a system using a simple series of exercises and posture positioning to prevent or relieve headaches, neck and shoulder pain, carpal tunnel syndrome, and upper and lower back pain. "The human body is its own mechanic," Weisberg wrote. "If you take it in for a tune-up {using his program} it will repair and heal itself." His program also details modified movements tailored to the needs of senior citizens and children.

A second exercise-based program, known as the McKenzie Method, developed by New Zealand physical therapist Robin McKenzie, focuses on relieving back and neck pain using seven extension exercises and posture corrections. Each exercise session lasts about one minute and these sessions are recommended to be repeated up to a half-dozen times a day. "To remain pain-free for life, adopt good posture and perform the exercises," he advised in his 2001 book, *7 Steps To A Pain-Free Life.* More than 20,000 physical therapists, physicians and chiropractors worldwide have been trained in the McKenzie Method for use with their patients.

Chapter 11

Eight Natural, Effective Pain Relief Practices

Pain relief without using pharmaceutical drugs encompasses many different techniques and practices that have stood the test of time from repeated use without side effects, yet also have received an endorsement in more recent times from the 'gold standard' of medical science--- the peer-reviewed, placebo-controlled double-blind study.

I've singled out here eight easy, safe and effective approaches for you to try based on your pain relief needs. Experiment with what works for you. Create a healing synergy by combining two or more of these practices into a routine that fits into your lifestyle.

Here are the practices in alphabetical order.

(1) Cognitive Behavioral Therapy (CBT):
CBT capitalizes on the idea that your thoughts can both obstruct your ability to heal from physical or mental injury, or can enhance your capacity to heal. Usually working with a trained therapist, you are taught in an interactive process to identify negative or

irrational beliefs that hold you back from experiencing wellness.
It's a process that enables you to develop coping strategies based
on healthier thoughts, a variation on the 'mind over matter'
approach to combating pain.

Psychotherapist Donald Altman of Portland, Ore., uses CBT with
his patients, often in conjunction with mindfulness meditation,
and also promotes the practice in his various books, including *The
Mindfulness Code*. He explained how CBT works to help relieve
pain:

"CBT challenges distorted thoughts and beliefs. It works
to regulate emotions by having patients challenge the basis
for their emotional distress--and the underlying behaviors. It
increases understanding of primary emotions and understanding
of secondary emotions that are triggered by beliefs which increase
distress and pain. It helps people make the link between triggering
events and the thoughts, emotions, and behavior that follow. In
other words, you learn to trace the cause and effect pattern in your
mind that contributes to compulsive thoughts and behaviors that
trigger or intensify pain."

Here are a couple of studies illustrating the potential of CBT to
assist in relieving various types of painful conditions.

--Writing in an April 2006 issue of the journal, *Pain,* researchers
at the University of Washington School of Medicine documented
how CBT was effective in reducing chronic temporomandibular
disorder pain (this is the joint connecting the mandible to the
skull.) Compared to a control group, study participants in the CBT
group experienced three times higher levels of pain intensity relief.

--A February 2012 study in the *International Journal of Behavioral Medicine* examined CBT's effect on children suffering from chronic abdominal pain. A total of 29 children were randomly placed into two groups; a control group and an intervention group using CBT over six sessions. The outcome: "children in the intervention group experienced both a reduction in pain and an improvement in health-related quality of life compared to the control group. The effect sizes ranged from medium to high."

(2) Food (the good and the bad dietary practices):
You become what you eat, an old tried and tested cliché tells us, so if you eat nutritious foods and maintain a healthy diet, you cut your risks of illness, disease and their associated pains. If your diet consists of foods in conflict with your physical needs, you will trigger or worsen pain as a result of the unhealthy diet. It's that simple.

One of the pioneering studies showing a relationship between pain severity and diet was published in the British journal, *Lancet,* in October 1991, examining whether certain foods affect the inflammation associated with arthritis. Milk and eggs were two of the culprits identified as increasing pain and joint stiffness. Those patients in the study who avoided eating these foods showed dramatic improvement in their pain severity levels.

In his book, *Foods That Fight Pain,* Dr. Neal Barnard reviewed dozens of studies investigating the food and pain link. He identified meats, dairy products and eggs as major triggers for many types of pain, particularly joint pain associated with arthritis. Corn can also trigger pain symptoms in sensitive people. Natural anti-inflammatory painkillers include vegetables (broccoli, spinach, etc.), beans, fruits, and flaxseed oil, canola, wheat-germ, and walnut oils. Hot chili peppers contain capsaicin, which has been proven to help block the nerves' ability to send pain messages to the brain.

For aching joints and the pain of osteoarthritis, a series of studies found avocado/soybean oil extract to be an effective remedy. The suggested dosage amount is 300 milligrams a day. Medical writer Bill Gottlieb, in his 2008 book, *Breakthroughs in Drug-Free Healing,* presents many dozens of food-based pain cures that have been validated by medical studies., along with other non-food non-drug techniques for dealing with post-operative pain, fibromyalgia, back pain, migraines, and may other maladies.

Nutrients you can't normally get in sufficient quantities from your diet also can be pain fighters if taken in supplement form. Nutritional biochemist Shawn M. Talbott, Ph.D., recommends the following herbal preparations in his 2006 book, *Natural Solutions for Pain-Free Living:*
    ---For joint pain, the herbal combination of scutellaria and acacia.
    ---Muscle and soft tissue pain, try the anti-inflammatory herbal extracts boswellia, ginger, turmeric, avocado/soy extracts, or scutellaria.
    ---Arthritis and Osteoarthritis pain, consumer grape seed extract and green tea.

(3) Guided Imagery:
Another way to tap into the healing power of your mind for pain relief is by using your imagination to summon soothing images.

During a painful dental extraction, for instance, you could imagine an ocean beach, the rhythmic lapping of the waves, the feel of wet sand between your toes.

The state of relaxation entered during a visualization session resembles what can be achieved during meditation. During the 1980s and 90s a Buffalo, N.Y. dentist, Philip Ament, gained media attention for his use of visualization for pain control. Rather than full anesthesia, he used soothing images in which the patients visualized themselves becoming numb during dental surgery.

Imagery helps the body to release endorphins, the human body's natural pain-fighting chemicals, and it helps to trigger the placebo response, the power of suggestion, which is yet another of the natural healing resources we humans have been blessed with. A useful technique to incorporate with visualization is the mantra, the repetition of a word or phrase with special meaning for you, such as, "I am strong. I will not feel the pain."

Medical science evidence for the pain-fighting effectiveness of guided imagery has been rapidly accumulating over the past decade or so. In a May 1999 issue of *The Journal of Head and Face Pain,* for example, researchers did an experiment with 129 patients suffering from chronic tension-type headaches. The visualization intervention group reported "significantly more improvement" in all measurements of pain after each session and after one month of the guided imagery tape therapy.

A key to the success of visualization hinges on the person's ability not only to generate mental images, but to become absorbed in them as if they were real. A 2009 study in the *Journal of Psychiatric Research* monitored 55 women with previously diagnosed fibromyalgia pain. They were divided into two groups. One received relaxation training and guided instruction in how to generate pleasant imagery in order to distract themselves from the pain. A control group received treatment as usual. Concluded the study authors: "Pleasant imagery was an effective intervention in reducing fibromyalgic pain during the 28-day study period."

Finally, from among many dozens of studies showing the beneficial effects on pain, here is one conducted with a group of 30 senior citizens suffering from osteoarthritis pain. Published in a March 2010 issue of *Pain Management Nursing,* this four-month clinical trial of guided imagery found that the process reduced pain levels and lowered prescribed arthritis medication use. The study authors urged pain management physicians to incorporate guided imagery in their toolbox of treatments.

(4) Hypnosis:
This relaxation system strives to control the brain's reactions, thoughts or perceptions. A person can also try to control his or her own brain process through "self-hypnosis."

Practitioners of hypnosis claim that for the most part people who willingly get hypnotized often respond readily to suggestions— either physically or psychologically. While the process is actually quite complex, hypnotists strive verbally and non-verbally to focus the person's conscious mind on a single predominant objective or idea in order to make the individual more susceptible to suggestions. Battling pain can be among this system's potential goals.

At a Belgian hospital, Cliniques Universitaires St. Luc in Brussels, physicians use hypnosis on patients before their surgeries to reduce their need for painkillers and to accelerate their recovery time. A July 27, 2011 Associated Press article about the practice noted: "Doctors say nearly any surgery usually done with a local anesthetic could work with hypnosis and less pain medicine. Proponents say hypnosis can dull patients' sense of pain and that it also cuts down on the need for anesthetic. Since doctors began offering hypnosis at the hospital in 2003, hundreds of patients have chosen it."

The article described how a 43-year-old woman had her thyroid surgically removed while under hypnosis. She pictured herself hiking in the mountains as surgeons did the operation. Breast cancer surgeries, including mastectomies and biopsies, commonly use hypnosis at this hospital.

Quite a few medical studies have affirmed the usefulness of hypnosis in fighting pain. The *International Journal of Clinical & Experimental Hypnosis* featured a study in January 2011 that tested the effects of self-hypnosis on individuals with multiple sclerosis and chronic pain. The University of Washington researchers concluded that their findings "supported the greater beneficial effects of self-hypnosis training on average pain intensity."

Writing in the *Journal of Pain,* five Spanish scientists in January 2012 published the results of their study of fibromyalgia patients and hypnosis combined with Cognitive-Behavioral Group Therapy. Ninety-three fibromyalgia patients were randomly assigned to one of three experimental groups. The group using hypnosis and therapy had far better outcomes than the other groups on pain severity measurement scales.

(5) Massage (and therapeutic touch):
Getting a massage, as anyone who has had one already knows, relieves tension and reduces the intensity of most types of pain. "Past studies have managed to show only that a well-administered rub can reduce pain, but none has ever pinpointed how," observed a February 1, 2012 article in *Science* magazine.

As the magazine went on to note, that mystery has been partially solved thanks to research by Canadian scientists who found that massages reduce the levels of a chemical in the body which turns on genes association with inflammation. "There's no question I'm going to be visiting the massage therapist more often," quipped one of the study authors, Dr. Mark Tarnopolsky from McMaster University in Hamilton, Canada.

Therapeutic touch to ease pain is also something you can perform on yourself, without the assistance of a massage therapist. That was the conclusion of a September 2010 study published in *Current Biology*, in which British and French scientists subjected a group of volunteers to pain perception tests using fingers and various temperatures of water.

When the lab volunteers touched fingers of one hand to fingers of another hand dipped in painful heated water, pain levels dropped 64 percent compared to levels without self-touch being administered. The research team concluded that levels of acute pain not only depend on signals sent to the brain, but also rely on how the human brain "integrates these signals into a coherent representation of the body as a whole" In other words, any therapy such as massage and self-touch has the potential to reduce pain because it assists the brain in shaping the experience in beneficial ways we never suspected before.

We know that healing touch has a long history in the human experience. The New Testament of the Bible describes Jesus using the 'laying on of hands' to heal people in pain. This tradition developed in many diverse cultures and continues up through the present day.

Some of the early modern research findings about touch and pain occurred in the 1980s. Chronic back pain was the subject of an experiment by Dr. Michael Weintraub, chief of neurology at Phelps Memorial Hospital in New York City. He had 63 of his patients with chronic pain undergo twice weekly shiatsu-style massages---more than three-fourths of the patients achieved significant pain relief from their chronic back conditions.

Pain associated with cancer was assessed in a University of South Carolina experiment conducted by two Ph.D.'s, Sally Weinrich and Martin Weinrich. They placed 28 cancer patients in two groups---one group got ten-minute massages, the other group only a ten-minute visit. Pain level measurement determined that pain levels decreased for all patients receiving the massages.

(6) Meditation (also combined with forgiveness):
Embracing traditions and methods used for thousands of years, people who meditate practice to rid their minds of thoughts and any awareness of sensations. Practitioners of meditation view the mind as a powerful force capable of focusing upon or ignoring physical or mental sensations.

Those who meditate use a variety of methods to achieve the

mental state they seek, such as the concentration on compassionate thoughts or repeating a mantra (a series of words.) Many branches of meditation stem from ancient Eastern religions or traditions such as Buddhism or Hinduism.

In his 2011 book *Natural Pain Relief: How to Soothe & Dissolve Physical Pain with Mindfulness,* meditation teacher Shinzen Young describes exercises to 'retrain' your relationship to pain using traditional meditation practices, particularly the technique called mindfulness meditation. (An hour-long CD is included with the book providing guided meditations for pain.) "The underlying theme of Mindfulness Meditation is the concept of 'divide and conquer,'" writes Young. "If an experience is overwhelming you, break it into its parts, and keep track of them as they arise moment by moment. Often the separate parts are quite manageable individually, hence the aggregate experience loses its power to overwhelm you." He goes on to detail how you can use the power of observation and your breathing to divide pain sensations based on separating the thoughts, emotions, and actual physical feelings until you can actually manage pain to be more bearable.

It's well known that anxiety and stress can increase pain intensity. So anything that naturally decreases anxiety and stress automatically has potentially beneficial effects on pain symptoms. Meditation helps to break the shackles of pain, as countless studies have demonstrated. For example, meditation techniques have been a staple course of teaching at Stanford University's arthritis self-help program with documented positive results in reducing arthritic pain.

If you add feelings of 'loving-kindness' or a practice of forgiveness to a meditation technique, you actually increase the benefits related to pain management. That's been the finding of numerous studies. Here are just two examples.

At Duke University Medical Center, a team of seven researchers used a loving-kindness meditation, designed to transform anger into compassion, with 43 patients suffering from chronic low back pain. The program lasted eight weeks. Results published in a September 2005 issue of the *Journal of Holistic Nursing* confirmed "significant improvements in pain and psychological distress" among those in the loving-kindness group. By letting go of resentments and anger associated with traumas, people or events, pain sufferers are better able to cope with pain because they have released the triggers that intensify pain.

Finally, in a landmark study published during February 2005 in the *Journal of Pain,* researchers studies another 61 patients with chronic low back pain and concluded that "Clinical observations suggest that many patients with chronic pain have difficulty forgiving persons they perceive as having unjustly offended them in some way…patients who had higher scores on forgiveness-related variables reported lower levels of pain, anger and psychological distress…this study suggests there is a relationship between forgiveness and pain."

(7) Music Therapy:
We all know that music can be a source of relaxation and pleasure, irrespective of one's musical tastes. There is evidence, however, that when it comes to using music to help relieve pain, you need to emphasize melodies that soothe and calm you, not arouse you.

That is why classical music generally works better than most kinds of contemporary tunes.

Consider some of the study evidence for the role that music can play. A December 2011 study published in the journal, *Clinical Rheumatology*, placed 62 patients undergoing joint lavage for knee osteoarthritis into one of two groups---a control group receiving no music intervention, and an intervention group listening to recorded music. The median age was 68 years old and two-thirds of the study participants were women. The findings were unequivocal: "Music is a simple and effective tool to alleviate pain and anxiety in patients undergoing joint lavage for knee osteoarthritis."

Another study in an April 2011 issue of *The Journal of Clinical Nursing* evaluated the effects of music therapy on 60 patients receiving spine surgery. The study group participants listened to selected music from the evening before their surgery through the second day after the surgery was performed. Once again, the findings were clear: "Music therapy can alleviate pain and anxiety in patients before and after spinal surgery."

To evaluate the effects of music on pain levels in cancer patients, researchers examined 30 clinical trials conducted on 1,891 cancer patients and published their results in an August 2011 issue of *Cochrane Database System Review*. In 17 of the studies examined the patients listened to prerecorded music, while in the remaining studies they actually took part in guided music therapies with song, piano playing or other expressions. The researchers' conclusion: "this systematic review indicates that music interventions may have beneficial effects on anxiety, pain, mood and quality of life in people with cancer."

French scientists writing in *The Clinical Journal of Pain,* October 2011, used music with 87 patients afflicted with lumbar pain, fibromyalgia, inflammatory disease or neurological disease. They received at least two daily sessions of music and on returning home from the hospital, continued the music intervention. "This music intervention method appears to be useful in managing chronic pain as it enables a significant reduction in the consumption of medication," the research team concluded.

Most of us parents have seen music work in practice with our children. That's why lullabies exist for kids, to calm them down and distract them from anxiety or pain. Music is a low-cost, no side effects type of intervention that pain patients can control by selecting their own 'dosage' levels and style of therapy. If one style of music isn't working well, you can always switch the channel or pull out another type of music for easy listening.

(8) Yoga:
There are a lot of misconceptions about what yoga is and isn't when practiced outside of India, where it originated. Yoga isn't a religion, though it developed from Hinduism, and yoga isn't just a form of exercise, though it does involve a lot of stretching and movement.

The emphasis in yoga is on posture and breath control. Sometimes meditation is incorporated at the beginning or end of yoga sessions. There are at least six different types of yoga being practiced and one of the most popular is Iyengar yoga, named after B.K.S. Iyengar, whose yoga training clinic in India draws thousands of Western practitioners. This yoga practice puts a lot of attention on holding a posture/position (an asana) and slowly deepening it.

Much of the research on the clinical potential of yoga to soothe pain has occurred only in the last decade. An October 2011 study in the *Archives of Internal Medicine*, for instance, examined 228 healthy adults with moderate chronic back pain. They were randomly assigned to one of three study groups. One took weekly 75-minute yoga classes, the second group did stretching exercises, while the third just read a book on back pain. Both yoga and stretching flexibility exercises produced an improvement in back pain resulting in a decreased use of medication.

Additional evidence for yoga's benefits came from a July 2011 study in the *Journal of Pain Research* in which Canadian scientists determined that practicing yoga reduces symptoms of chronic pain in women with fibromyalgia. The participants did a program of 75 minutes of hatha yoga twice weekly over a period of eight weeks that the study went on. It was the first study to evaluate the effect of yoga on elevating cortisol levels in the body, which seems to be the natural chemical mechanism by which pain is reduced following a yoga workout.

"Yoga promotes this concept that we are not our bodies, our experiences, or our pain. This is extremely useful in the management of pain," said study co-author Kathryn Curtis in a media commentary released by York University. "We saw their levels of mindfulness increase—they were better able to detach from their psychological experience of pain. Our findings strongly suggest that psychological changes in turn affect our experience of physical pain."

Chapter 12

"Medical" Marijuana Can Be A Pain Killer

Medical evidence has been accumulating for the past decade that marijuana can be a safe and effective treatment for some forms of chronic pain, either as a substitute for pharmaceutical drugs, or when used in combination with other painkillers.

As one illustration, a December 2011 study published in *Clinical Pharmacology and Therapeutics* reported how 21 men and women suffering from a range of conditions—arthritis, cancer, multiple sclerosis—inhaled vaporized marijuana three times a day. They were already taking daily doses of either morphine or oxycodone to treat their chronic pain.

What occurred was a 'synergistic' therapeutic effect (cannabis and the opiates together produced pain relief effects much greater than any one substance did on its own.) Overall, study participants achieved a 25 percent additional reduction in their pain index levels from this drug combination.

Keep in mind the study participants were experiencing severe chronic pain from their medical conditions, so the therapeutic use of marijuana, according to the study authors, provides hope "that marijuana could someday be used as a replacement for narcotics to help curb some of the side effects associations with those medications."

This study added more evidence weight to dozens of previous medical studies demonstrating the pain reduction potential of the two main compounds of marijuana—cannabidiol (CBD) and delta-9 tetrahydrocannabinol (THC). A drug called Sativex, already being used in Europe, combines these two compounds for treatment of pain in cancer patients, and awaits clinical trials in the U.S.

The super-charged, highly emotional issue of whether marijuana should be used in treating pain and illness erupted across the American political landscape during the final decades of the 20th Century and into the 21st.

Needless to say, this issue steadily evolved into perhaps the most hotly debated choice involving the treatment of pain, taking much of the spotlight in the mainstream media. To say that "weed," "grass" or "smokes" are harmless sparks the ire of people who swear that such treatments are merely an excuse for getting high.

Advocates of such treatments, the people who argue that such systems should get legitimized worldwide, insist that smoking or eating marijuana is highly effective in the treatment of chemotherapy, AIDS, nausea, vomiting, anorexia, pain and other ailments.

Who benefits from keeping marijuana illegal?" asked George Soros, a Hungarian-American financier, philanthropist and businessman. "The greatest beneficiaries are the criminal organizations in Mexico, and elsewhere that earn billions of dollars annually from this illicit trade—and who would rapidly lose their competitive advantage if marijuana were a legal commodity."

Like opium and willow tree bark, the active ingredient in marijuana beneficial in fighting pain grows in nature—but in this case as a "weed." Labeled by the United Nations as the "most widely used illicit substance in the world," the cannabis plant creates a powerful psychoactive chemical compound commonly known as THC.

Biologists believe that marijuana, known to some researchers as "cannabis," naturally developed THC as a defensive mechanism, perhaps to fight off herbivores or organisms that eat plants. According to a 2009 article in *Archives of General Psychiatry*, a whopping 400 different chemical compounds are in cannabis.

Archaeological research indicates that some people began using marijuana as far back as 3,000 years before Christ. Cannabis use occurred thousands of years ago in such diverse places as China, Bulgaria, Greece and early Iran. Whether these early cultures used marijuana to kill or block pain remains a matter of dispute.

Although marijuana is much less powerful than opium and opiate-based drugs, various countries began to criminalize cannabis through the early 1900s including New Zealand, the United Kingdom, Jamaica and South Africa. In 1906, authorities in

Washington, D.C., imposed restrictions on cannabis, and the U.S. Congress passed the "Marihuana Tax Act," placing a tax on the sale of cannabis, while prohibiting the production of marijuana and its byproduct, hemp.

Although the use of marijuana for medicinal purposes remains controversial, one can't ignore the fact that numerous studies cite its effectiveness as an analgesic or pain reliever, according to various medical studies. Researchers also insist that their studies indicate the effectiveness of cannabis in treating glaucoma, and AIDS—while also stimulating hunger in cancer patients as they undergo chemotherapy.

Despite such findings, the U.S. Food and Drug Administration hasn't authorized the use of marijuana for medical purposes. Meantime, a federal law enforcement agency, the Drug Enforcement Administration or DEA pursues those who distribute or produce marijuana with the same ferocity as "heavy" drugs like heroin and cocaine.

"Penalties against possession of a drug should not be more damaging to an individual than the use of the drug itself, and where they are they should be charged," said Jimmy Carter, 39th president of the United States. Despite such political convictions, the severity and potential harmfulness remains a matter of dispute involving specific drug types—especially marijuana.

Cannabis can be administered in a variety of methods, most often smoking, inhaling or eating when baked into common foods such as brownies. Meantime, while the use of marijuana for medical purposes remains a highly disputed hot political topic, such activities are deemed legally permissible in only a limited number of countries and states.

Fighting Pain with Marijuana Is a Moral Choice

The question of whether to use marijuana in medicine remains a hot moral issue as people argue sharply diverse opinions. Yet society needs to realize that literally all highly powerful pain killing medications remain extremely powerful and potentially dangerous, not just cannabis.

By recent accounts, the use of marijuana via prescription for legitimate medical purposes is allowed in varying degrees in at least 16 states including California, by far the most populous of them. And, the Golden State is among seven that authorize dispensaries for medically prescribed cannabis; the others are Michigan, Montana, Rhode Island, Maine, New Mexico and Colorado.

Complicating matters, however, marijuana remains an illegal drug and the federal Food and Drug Administration has issued a controversial advisory stating that while marijuana is subject to abuse, there is "no currently accepted medical use (of marijuana) in treatment in the United States." According to some published reports, the only instance where the FDA authorizes the medical use of cannabis is in oral form as dronabinol or nabilone. These are sometimes used only after other standard treatments fail to work in alleviating adverse symptoms such as nausea and vomiting associated with chemotherapy.

Paradoxically, the sale of marijuana still remains illegal under federal law, even in the wake of a 2009 U.S. Justice Department memo to all state attorneys general. The document provided seven criteria that prosecutors can use when determining to pursue criminal action in specific medical marijuana cases. At the same time, though, federal officials recommended against prosecuting patients who have followed state laws in receiving and using such prescriptions.

One of the most common criticisms stemmed from concerns that the process of smoking cannabis would threaten the patients' health. Advocates of such treatments insist that doctors have managed to efficiently and legally sidestep such concerns thanks to much safer consumption methods such as inhaling marijuana aroma processed through a vaporizer, or when eating THC-laden food.

Willie Nelson, a popular American musician and entertainer, has been quoted as saying that "I think people need to be educated to the fact that marijuana is not a drug. Marijuana is an herb and a flower. God put it here. If he put it here and he wants it to grow, what gives the government the right to say that God is wrong?"

On the so-called flip side of this proverbial coin, though, some law enforcement officials still insist that marijuana even for medical use is a "doorway drug," opening up the possibility that an individual will become addicted to much more harmful substances.

Weigh the Facts Before Using Medical Marijuana

From my personal and professional view, many people fake illnesses or seek phony cannabis prescriptions just so they can abuse marijuana as a recreational drug. Overall, this stems from the same potentially harmful process that lots of consumers use to obtain extremely harmful and dangerously addictive pain-killing drugs produced by pharmaceutical companies and dispersed by local pharmacies.

Ultimately, the decision on whether to legally use marijuana for medical reasons should not be taken lightly by patients or physicians. Doctors have a moral and professional responsibility to only prescribe drugs for legitimate and useful reasons as medical treatments.

With this in mind, I recommend that patients pursuing or considering the possibility of marijuana prescriptions to take the following precautions at the very least:

- **Prognosis:** Is your current medical condition or pain truly significant, to the point where you would want to even consider using such a substance?

- **Alternatives:** Before pursuing or even considering such a prescription, patients should study the possibility of other more traditional medications, herbs or lifestyles. An oral prescription form of THC is available for patients suffering from nausea, vomiting and anorexia.

- **Reputation:** Study the background, education and overall reputation of the physician who might prescribe marijuana for you. Does he or she have a good reputation for issuing such treatments only in specific, essential instances?

- **Cost:** Some patients, especially those with low incomes, also might feel a need to research potential costs for marijuana prescriptions. Be sure to check whether your insurance company covers the cost of such drugs. And, if not, you should ponder whether the potential benefit would be worth the expense.

- **Abuse:** As a physician, I always recommend that patients strive to avoid abusing drugs of any kind ranging from alcohol to highly illegal narcotics. Anyone striving to obtain such a prescription merely in order to abuse marijuana should seek to get professional help, either by first inquiring with a physician or visiting organizations such as Narcotics Anonymous.

While approaching this possibility from a serious and thoughtful perspective, some patients also might want to keep in mind that serious research has indicated the medical use of marijuana generates definite benefits—at least in some specific instances.

A 2009 article in the *Journal of Clinical Investigation* said that in some studies marijuana use was effective in killing harmful brain cancer cells while leaving healthy cells intact within the organ. Another 2009 article on PhysOrg.com cited a study concluding that stressed rats injected with the THC byproduct of cannabis became less dependant on opiates. And according to media reports at least one other study indicated the apparent effectiveness of marijuana in lessening the muscular spasms and swelling sometimes suffered by people with multiple sclerosis.

When referring to marijuana, the late Nobel Prize-winning economist and statistician of the 20th Century, Milton Friedman, said, "When a private enterprise fails, it is closed down; when a government enterprise fails, it is expanded. Isn't that exactly what is happening with drugs?"

The newest member of the marijuana family is so-called "hemp oil," which has less psychoactive activity and more anti-cancer activity. This product is currently under invesigative research at UC San Francisco Department of Integrative Oncology.

Chapter 13

The Future of Pain Relief

As described in my book *Anti-Aging Cures*, natural human growth hormones are an effective way to slow down the signs of aging—and for speeding up the natural healing process as well.

For those who have not yet read my book, in summary, human growth hormone (HGH) is produced within the brain. This sparks the continual growth process in children, progressing until their early adult years in their mid-20s. After that age, the body's natural production of HGH steadily slows and people begin to show the signs of aging, such as wrinkles, weight gain and the weakening of bones.

When we're young, though, high levels of HGH that are bodies naturally generate, most often while we sleep, enable us to recover and heal rapidly from wounds and broken bones. Yet older people generally do not recover from such maladies as quickly as the very young, primarily due to the body's steady decrease in production of the hormone after age 25.

This is where the controversy erupts. You see, much of the general public wrongly believes that HGH is illegal. To the contrary, within the United States, the substance is legal when prescribed by a certified medical professional after first conducting a physical examination.

When used properly, HGH can go a long way toward rapidly speeding up the healing process and thereby removing pain—even among our younger wounded soldiers who already naturally produce the hormone at a fairly strong pace. The misconception about HGH stems largely from its use in professional sports. Journalists often give HGH an unnecessary and unwarranted bad rap.

Make HGH More Widely Accessible

To heal wounds faster and thereby accelerate the natural decrease in pain, hospital emergency rooms nationwide and around the world need to make HGH more readily available to victims of accidents and extreme trauma such as gunshot wounds.

Since HGH reigns as a naturally occurring and vital biological substance, administering this hormone under proper conditions at recommended doses—but not in excessive amounts—should evolve into a preferred and logical alternative. This should become an accepted, logical potential alternative to some unnatural, highly dangerous and expensive medications that generate giant profits for "Big Pharma," the large pharmaceutical companies.

As a licensed homeopath and a seasoned oncologist and physician, I have witnessed many instances where standard, mainstream doctors ignore the natural substances such as HGH—even though this hormone can go a long way in the battle of fighting pain.

Sadly, however, many standard allopathic doctors are trained to do only what they're taught, which often means avoiding any natural treatments that would enable patients to heal the way that nature intended.

As a society, our entire culture needs to do more to accept and generate natural substances such as HGH, largely because they're far less expensive than many high-end pharmaceuticals while often proving more effective than potentially dangerous drugs issued and promoted by Big Pharma.

The Human Genome Project Offers Hope

Although science still lacks a significant, comprehensive "cure-all" for pain, researchers assisted by physicians and medical experts have made tremendous progress in recent decades.

Much of this success stems from the Human Genome Project, in which scientists have mapped all 20,000-25,000 genes in our bodies. The bulk of this initial work occurred from 1987 to 2003, when scientists announced that they had chronicled or recorded all basic gene structures that operate the body's physical and functional systems.

For many generations to come, medical professionals and physicians will likely use this vital information in developing essential treatments and drugs for a wide variety of specific conditions. Pain likely will become a prime target of these efforts.

According to various medical journals and news reports, experts reviewing and studying the project's massive database already have determined that hereditary genetics often play a role in passing the tendency for pain to subsequent generations. Just as compelling, some individuals apparently have a predisposition to certain types of pain.

Adding even more questions to the complex mysteries of the human body, researchers also report that they have found that some individuals also inherit an inclination for inflammation and perhaps even tendencies for excessive or chronic pain.

These general findings come as no surprise to medical historians who point out that in 1866 the monk Gregor Mendel discovered that common peas displayed characteristics of inherited traits. Along with James D. Watson, in the 20th Century a British biologist and neurologist, Francis Crick used Mendel's research as the basis for their own Nobel Prize-winning discovery that the double helix of genes forms a primary basis of life.

The term "double helix" is used in molecular biology to describe double-stranded molecules that form DNA—scientifically called Deoxyribonucleic acid—a nucleic acid that contains genetic instructions for the basis of life. The double helix phenomenon also plays a significant role in RNA—Ribonucleic acid—a macromolecule deemed necessary in order for all known forms of life to exist.

Through much of the 20th Century, scientists used the findings of Watson and Crick as the basis for significant discoveries in a wide variety of crippling or fatal diseases. These painful maladies include breast cancer, cystic fibrosis, Down's syndrome, and many other debilitating conditions.

Buoyed by these numerous medical advances, scientists are working to delve much deeper into individual paired chromosomes in order to determine how to eliminate pain. In order to do this with any effectiveness, at least from my personal view, researchers will need to continue their ongoing and relentless efforts to methodically review and analyze each building block of the entire Human Genome Structure.

Look For Significant Progress Every Day

Without letup, researchers that you probably never heard about are keeping busy going step-by-step in methodically reviewing and analyzing each of the four primary building compounds of life—largely in an effort to identify and essentially wipe out the ravages of physical pain. These basic compounds are:

- **Adenine:** Serving as a chemical component of both DNA and RNA, adenine plays a variety of significant roles including cellular respiration, essential metabolic reactions and processes within cells in order to convert nutrients into energy.

- **Guanine:** Derived from purine, an organic compound, guanine plays a critical role in the formation of the double-bonded ring systems of both DNA and RNA.

- **Cytosine**: In the base pairing bond discovered by Watson and Crick, cytosine serves as the basis in the formation of guanine's three hydrogen bonds.

- **Thymine:** Scientists say this plays a critical role in stabilizing nucleic acid, a basic and necessary part of both DNA and RNA.

Following the rules or requirements of the human genome structure as mandated by Mother Nature, these four purine-based building blocks form a wide array of complex sequences. These, in turn, form an integral series of codes, building blocks for the master plan that makes each person unique and functional—plus how we feel and react to pain.

Key Triggers of Pain Will be Tricky To Isolate

For scientists and physicians seeking to eradicate physical pain, the key to success hinges largely on identifying specific points that trigger the signals of such symptoms. Among these, the most essential characteristics are commonly called SNPs, referred to by physicians as "single nucleotide polymorphisms." This factor remains highly critical, primarily because SNPs can produce subtle variations in the manner in which separate individuals respond to specific illnesses, injuries or various forms of trauma.

Besides regulating or signaling varying responses to pain, the SNP system and process also plays a significant dual role in determining, regulating and managing how our cells respond, absorb and react to drugs, food and essential nutrients such as vitamins.

Needless to say, as a result of these highly complex and interdependent processes, physicians and medical professionals are now faced with a formidable task. The key to success hinges on creating medical strategies to effectively balance these various factors, essentially an integral and difficult-to-achieve balancing act.

"Being on a tightrope is living, everything else is waiting," said Karl Wallenda, the famed founder of the popular Flying Wallendas daredevil circus act of the 20th Century. Wallenda died in 1978 at age 73 when he fell from a tightrope 121 feet above ground between two towers in San Juan, Puerto Rico.

Yes, in a sense, while working diligently to generate effective pain remedies, researchers of the human genome structure are essentially walking a tightrope. But unlike the sturdy and predictable ropes or wires that Wallenda walked, the subtle variations within the gene map of the human body can unexpectedly sway or move in unpredictable ways.

Herein rests the key to success, continually refining and fine-tuning our potential abilities to manage or isolate gene structures that regulate everything from swelling, stress, inflammation, detoxification and a vast array of other bodily functions.

Despite these many formidable challenges, scientists should proceed with enthusiasm and careful due diligence in actively pursuing these hoped-for solutions. After all, as the late movie star James Dean once said, "Dream as if you'll live forever, live as if you'll die today."

Discover Your Unique DNA Characteristics

With continued progress, individual consumers hopefully will someday be able to receive a comprehensive analysis of their own personal, individual gene structures.

On a comprehensive level, this would enable a person to determine his or her own propensity toward swelling, specific types of pain, abilities to detoxify, limit inflammation, and a wide array of other necessary bodily functions.

As the old saying promises, "knowledge is power." But even more important from the perspective of those eager to reduce pain, the ability to get an individualized DNA map could open up doors leading to significant physical recovery. Such intricate discoveries might tend to infuriate huge pharmaceutical companies that profit from the propensity of consumers taking ineffective drugs or who undergo unhelpful treatment regimens.

"Every great advance in natural knowledge has involved the absolute rejection of authority," said Henry Thomas Huxley, a 19th Century English biologist known as "Darwin's Bulldog" for advocating Charles Darwin's theory of evolution.

When the time finally comes for each of us to acquire our personalized DNA maps in a private, accurate manner, we all should eagerly seek this essential information. Particularly those of us suffering from extensive physical pain should be able to look to such data as a guide or roadmap on how we can best manage our personal lifestyle behaviors. The gene map has already become critical for chemo-sensitivity testing of cancer patients.

For instance, a person who discovers from his personalized DNA map that he has a propensity to suffer from excessive swelling in certain joints, could modify his exercise routine in order to prevent or alleviate the probability of suffering such pain. Depending on the specific afflictions identified, potential ways to prevent or lessen pain could range from the consumption or avoidance of certain foods to the active exercise of certain muscle groups.

Take Decisive Action When Battling Your Pain

Every week patients from around the world visit my West Coast clinic in the United States to continue their battles against cancer and other physically painful conditions.

I encourage them to ask me as many questions as possible about the many potential ways to eliminate or lessen their bodily discomforts. Many want to know more about the natural alternatives, while others prefer to focus on so-called mainstream options. For each patient, of course, I only make recommendations or issue prescriptions and treatments after conducting a thorough medical examination and reaching a prognosis.

Perhaps my popularity among patients stems largely from word-of-mouth, such as those video proclamations many of them have made for my Website—DrForsythe.com. And, of course, I'm told that the increasing popularity of my books and those written about me play a huge role in attracting patients.

Many of my patients and work associates tell me they're amazed at my continued stamina although I'm now edging into my mid-70s. Unlike many successful doctors who only work three or four days weekly during the final stage of their careers, I work a minimum of five days weekly and sometimes much more. The stream of new patients at my clinic has intensified and increased markedly in recent years. All along, my drive and passion for the medical profession continues to blossom and increase more than ever before.

Maybe this stems in part from the fact that I practice what I preach, so to speak. And I exercise and eat healthy foods for the most part, a process that I recommend for all my patients in order to achieve or maintain good health—the desired physical condition that goes a long way in preventing painful diseases or injuries. In addition, I take daily supplements for my heart, prostate, cholesterol and immune system to fortify myself.

Ask Lots of Questions and Find the Right Doctors

Anyone suffering from extreme pain, or their conscious and caring relatives, should ask as many questions as possible when interacting with their doctors or medical professionals. You should always ask why specific procedures or medications are recommended, and for details on potential adverse side effects.

Just as important, remember to inquire about any viable natural alternatives, and even if such substances are possible to deaden severe pain without your having to resort to powerful, highly addictive opium-based pharmaceuticals.
Also, remember that when dealing solely with mainstream

physicians, you're likely to hear that natural healing methods or alternative medicines are nothing but "quackery." All along, even if given such negative statements, you should remain inquisitive and keep an open mind about your options.

From my way of thinking, if any mainstream doctor ever tells you that there is no hope for eliminating your physical pain other than via extremely dangerous drugs, you should actively seek or consider a variety of other options as well.

Certainly, no person should have to endure chronic physical pain, especially if such a condition might prevent you from enjoying at least a basic, sensible and fairly good quality of life. Ultimately, there are numerous highly effective options that you can always seek, but keep in mind that such remedies should be sought under the continual monitoring and guidance of a licensed medical professional.

You don't have to be a prisoner of pain or addictive pain killers any longer. Put the advice in this book to good use and free yourself from the bondage that pain so mercilessly inflicts.

About the Author

James W. Forsythe, M.D., H.M.D., is an author, anti-aging physician, and integrative medical oncologist specializing in the use of human growth hormone to combat the symptoms of aging. A native of Detroit, Michigan, Forsythe has won widespread acclaim for his many medical achievements in the battles against cancer. Details on Doctor Forsythe's medical practice and on his numerous books can be found at his Website, DrForsythe.com

CPSIA information can be obtained
at www.ICGtesting.com
Printed in the USA
LVOW10s0321250518
578492LV00022B/822/P